LEADING CHANGE
IN
HEALTHCARE

Empowering Leadership to Doctors and
Healthcare Professionals

Dr Pallavi Hoskote

MBBS, MBA, PGDip. Psychiatry

Director, MEDILEADERS

Clever Fox
PUBLISHING

Chennai • Bangalore

CLEVER FOX PUBLISHING
Chennai, India

Published by CLEVER FOX PUBLISHING 2023
Copyright © Dr Pallavi Hoskote 2023

All Rights Reserved.
ISBN: 978-93-56483-53-8

Author's Note

*T*he Indian healthcare industry is rapidly growing in leaps and bounds. To be a competent doctor in today's era, one needs to harness leadership skills. Being a good clinician is only one side of the coin. One must be a great team player, manage a practice, make informed decisions regarding one's career choice, become self-aware of one's strengths and weaknesses, make the right therapeutic decisions and have an outstanding work-life balance.

Healthcare is growing phenomenally. There is a dire need to bring vital leadership roles amongst healthcare providers and healthcare professionals so that they come up with innovative ideas to handle the current situation in the healthcare industry.

It must be agreed upon that the medical profession is like no other. It comes with a great passion for the subject and the desire to serve and make a difference; it also comes with its own hurdles, sacrifices and challenges.

Doctors occupying every single position in the public and private sectors have gone through many years of struggle and hard work to reach where they are today. It's all about conscious choices and how we cope with them.

Remember, good leaders are also good followers, working in teams. It's never wrong to put forth your ideas and thoughts depending on the situation; it is never wrong to listen to or follow suggestions if it is beneficial to the team and self in a positive way. Most importantly, it is not wrong during your training years to say, "I do not know" or "I do not understand", get your doubts cleared and be open to learning and relearning throughout your journey.

From the earlier part of medical school, medicos tend to develop habits such as long study hours or untimely eating habits. Young budding doctors put up with exam stress and cope with pressures from peers and their mentors. As professionals, work schedules and duties are erratic; working under specific management, within teams, or, for that matter, being a shareholder in a healthcare establishment or maintaining a clinic; all require one to have the right management skills and leadership skills to excel.

This endeavour here is to help doctors inculcate leadership values in their chosen profession, which is crucial in the given healthcare scenario. Instilling leadership behaviours in the initial stages of the journey in the medical field will help one become confident, empower themselves and empower others in turn.

There are enough materials, books and discussions available on healthcare leadership on all platforms, and it is easy to access, but something compact and exclusive to the doctor community was missing. Something that was a quick read as doctors lack the luxury of time, something that may introduce young budding doctors and medical professionals to the concepts of leadership.

My only hope is that doctors can be inspired to identify and not shy away from their strengths, work on overcoming their weaknesses, do exemplary work to make that difference for humanity and most importantly, take care of their own personal, physical and emotional well-being.

The important thing here is, when I speak of leadership, do not assume it to be limited to people who hold formal or top lead roles. It is important to relate to it in your particular formal or informal position that you currently hold, to your responsibilities, and the particular situation, be it in life generally or at work place.

No particular leadership style is the right way. There is no right or wrong type of leadership style; it is essential to recognise what your true strengths and weaknesses are; to be able to overcome and utilise skillsets learnt in the chosen profession to make a difference and be able to sustain and coexist in harmony; building great healthy work atmospheres that will have excellent patient outcomes.

Always keep your physical and mental health, as you have a long journey to embark on, as most doctors tend to ignore their health and well-being as they work day after day caring for their patients.

Dr Pallavi Hoskote
MBBS, MBA Healthcare Management,
PGDip Psychiatry, Director MediLeaders.

God and the Doctor we alike adore

But only when in danger, not before;

The danger o'er, both are alike requited,

God is forgotten, and the Doctor slighted.

– Robert Owen

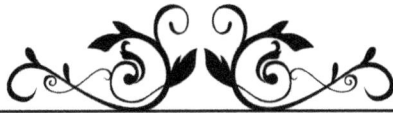

This book is dedicated to my love and life, may you always shine bright.

This book is for my family, friends, and every one of you reading this right now.

My dedication also goes to all the doctors and healthcare professionals of the past, present and future. You are all valuable, cherished and making a huge difference in people's lives every single day."

Dr Pallavi Hoskote
MBBS, MBA Healthcare Management,
PGDip Psychiatry, Director MediLeaders.

Index

"Only three things happen naturally in organisations: friction, confusion and underperformance. Everything else requires leadership"

– Peter Drucker

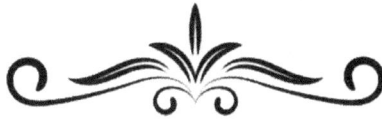

CHAPTER 1

INTRODUCTION

The present Indian Healthcare delivery basks complexity as most healthcare systems do. The healthcare sector is growing at a very fast pace. It is imperative at this time to consider and question if the healthcare managers, doctors, nurses and various healthcare professionals both in the public and the private sectors are ready to meet the ever-growing demands and strike a balance between new technologies, rapidly expanding health care industry and delivering patient centred quality care. And this calls for every individual in the healthcare industry, public or private to empower themselves and others with leadership behaviours, building strong healthcare organisations.

Research suggests that doctors make better managers, and indeed, better hospitals are the ones that are led by doctors. Known as the "heroic lone healers" at one time, doctors always had the quality of leadership hidden within them. The noble profession encompassing humanity needs to balance technological advances, challenging expectations and not to mention the added pressures doctors face working with the limited resources offered to them. To inculcate healthy work cultures calls for efficient and robust healthcare teams. The Indian healthcare system hence needs to see leadership in a new light, bringing much-needed transformation.

Background of the present healthcare system in India

The Ministry of Health and Family Welfare, state governments and local municipal bodies govern the Indian healthcare system. Every state has its own Department of Health, Health and Family Welfare Department and Directorate of Health. District-level health services oversee the primary care services; other agencies such as Insurance Regulatory and Development Authority regulate health insurance (Ministry of Health and Family Welfare, 2015). The healthcare system in India comprises both public and private sectors, delivering healthcare through complex networks; the healthcare delivery consists of three tiers which are the primary, secondary and tertiary healthcare facilities.

In rural India, primary healthcare delivery is through sub-centres, primary health centres and community health centres (Ministry of Health and Family Welfare, 2016). PHCs (primary health centres) cater to the village community through a medical officer. The community health centres are supported by specialist doctors, paramedics and other staff and should be equipped with beds and facilities like operating theatres and radiology equipment. The secondary and tertiary centres are located mainly in towns and cities. Doctors and healthcare professionals who work in government setups are paid fixed salaries and are not allowed to have their own private practice.

The private sector delivers most of the secondary, tertiary and quaternary care. The Indian healthcare industry is one of the largest sectors providing revenue and employment to people of different backgrounds. A large percentage of the population relies on the private sector for their healthcare needs. Private healthcare providers deliver outpatient and inpatient services through individual private clinics, small nursing homes, multispecialty clinics and small, medium-private and trust-run hospitals and corporate hospitals. The pay for doctors in the private sector depends on local market rates.

India, in recent times, has attracted medical tourism because it harbours a competent talent pool in the medical field, providing affordable healthcare compared to its Western and Asian counterparts. Health care in India has attracted investors from non-medical backgrounds and foreign investors.

Indian healthcare basks in complexity due to the presence of public and private sectors, the disparity in affordability and availability of services, technological advancements, competition between the private health caregivers, rising costs and challenges such as staff shortage.

Leadership and Healthcare

Until recently, leadership was only spoken about in the business sector. The challenge met while considering the leadership skills of healthcare professionals is that leadership theories were developed in the context of the business sector rather than within the healthcare arena.

While leadership in the business world involves power, profits, achievements and competition, the healthcare industry is different as it deals with life-the precious health of their customers (patients). Providing quality healthcare and a hassle-free experience on the road to recovery are strong backbones of any healthcare organisation or, for that matter, an essential mark of a great doctor.

In this new era of the healthcare industry, because of the involvement of corporate players, healthcare start-ups and entrepreneurs from varied backgrounds trying their hands at innovative healthcare delivery services through digitalisation, teleconsultations, app services, online healthcare services and not to mention small and sizeable private healthcare establishments, there is power, competition and profits involved. They need to sustain the health establishment and keep it going and doing good quality work, not to mention achievements in providing innovative advanced and safe treatments.

Many believe that leaders are the ones who set the backdrop, create context and that is definitely true. There are leaders who the people choose; for example, the CEO of a health organisation is appointed by the shareholders of that health establishment. There are also a few examples of doctors who have, on their own, built state-of-the-art healthcare establishments with their vision and the help of efficient teams.

It is critical for all doctors to possess leadership skills, to be able to create a domain for themselves, to recognise the challenges they may face in advance and to have forethought and plan accordingly. Leadership skills are not only required to achieve something or build or manage a health establishment, but it is also necessary to work and sustain in the current healthcare industry.

Doctors and healthcare professionals need to possess the reflective ability and should be able to choose from amongst various treatment options that are available to their patients, to be able to work in teams, take risky lifesaving decisions for the well-being of the patient or for that matter, be able to decide what kind of practice would be their strength. While some prefer and like working in the government sector, some prefer to work in a corporate hospital; the others wanting to set up their clinics or nursing homes and not mention those who want to go to another country to gain more expertise and choose to come back or practice outside their country.

Creating a healthy work atmosphere for oneself and others calls for leadership at every level of the healthcare echelon. One does not need a significant position to inculcate leadership skills, and it is not necessary that people who hold important positions are great leaders. The other way around is also true.

So, why is it essential for one to know about concepts of leadership or the theories behind it? I believe it is not to put oneself or fit oneself under any of those leadership types or styles and definitely not to attach oneself or mimic a type of leadership style. It is to be aware that such concepts and types exist and they may help one realise their weaknesses or strengths, so that they can work on the same and be able to thrive and do splendidly well in their chosen profession, or for that matter, understand themselves and live a fulfilling life.

History of Leadership

As Grint et al. (2011) asked, why bother about the history of leadership? Why bother about where it all started? Could we learn from history if it did repeat itself? To quote the most recent example, out of the blue, there was the COVID-19 pandemic. The Spanish flu and other pandemics gave our epidemiologists and scientists an insight to predict the course of the pandemic; scientific advancements have made humans get access to vaccines. Humans have been able to deal with this pandemic in a much more advanced manner. Hence, history does give us much-needed insight so that we can build and innovate as we advance into the future.

Even if history does not repeat itself, there may be patterns in the current day scenario that one can identify and predict as to what may or may not happen, helping us to strategise the course of action. However, it is also wise to remember that every situation is new and will come with its own challenges and will have unique never before attempted solutions, which goes to say that, with time, everything is evolving; there may be similarities but never the same challenge.

Leadership has existed since the time of human existence. Mostly, the knowledge of leadership in ancient times is dependent on the existence of written texts, such as that of Julius Caesar or Alexander The Great's victories and of emperor Ashoka's. It is quite clear that war was a critical factor in the early developments of leadership; from the Ramesses II of Egypt to the Harappan civilisation in the Indus Valley, military leadership played a role in domination and survival (Grint et al. 2011).

During 370 BC, Kautilya, through his visions for Chandra Gupta Maurya of the Mauryan dynasty, wrote a book called Arthasashtra, which listed the duties of a king, about utilising power and how to keep his subjects content; he spoke about administration, economy, financial management, leadership and governance (Grint et. al. 2011). Chanakya was a visionary and his Arthasashtra was so advanced that it holds good even today.

During Plato's time, he believed that education was an essential component to being a good leader and a leader works for the betterment of his people; he also acknowledged that a political system is necessary for leaders to emerge (Grint et al. 2011).

During the 19th century, Sigmund Freud of Germany suggested from his experience in psychoanalysis that leadership was an unconsciously exhibited behaviour. His theory talks about how the inner drivers influence the behaviour of an individual and that every neurotic symptom or action has an underlying reasoning; Further, his contemporaries applied the psychodynamic theory to workplace, suggesting that the early experiences of a leader influence his behaviour, and it shapes the functioning of the workplace and has an impact on the employees (Kets de Vries & Cheak, 2014).

Historically, in India, leadership was mostly identified with royalty or individuals in politics, finance, religion and culture. Leadership either came by birth or was inborn, while the rest could only admire and look up to. The history of leadership dates back to ancient times, mainly associated with mythology, royalty, ministry, religion and the affluent.

India's freedom struggle gave birth to countless heroes who led the country to its liberation.

Since the time India got its Independence, politics and leadership seemed to go synonymously with each other. There are entrepreneurs, industrialists, religious and spiritual leaders and not to mention the celebrities, sportsmen and artists who have a significant influence on society.

History of Leadership in Healthcare

Hospitals seem to have existed from ancient times in the Indian subcontinent. In the 6th century BC, the time of Gautama Buddha, there were many hospitals to look after the disabled and the ill; Charaka, the court physician of King Kanishka and Sushruta, the celebrated surgeon of his time, contributed to the field of medicine; numerous health establishments were opened throughout the country by Emperor Ashoka (273–232 BC); in the 16th century, European missionaries introduced the western Allopathic system of medicine to the country; the first of the hospitals were constructed during the British rule and organised medical training was initiated in the 19th century (Tabish, 2000).

When it comes to the history of leadership in healthcare, there are many examples of leaders who made a massive difference in the healthcare field. As cited by Sheingold and Hahn (2014), the history of quality in healthcare begins with Florence Nightingale; In 1854, when the British Troops fought the Russians to leave the Turkish territories, Cholera and diarrhoea were rampant, causing mortality amongst the British soldiers; Florence Nightingale was sent to Turkey and within the next six months, the mortality rate rapidly dropped; she concentrated on reducing overcrowding, making provision for ventilation, removing cavalry horses that were kept in the basement of the hospital and disinfecting the drains and latrines with peat charcoal (Nightingale, 1863). Nightingale documented that if the above steps had been followed, it would have prevented unnecessary mortality of the soldiers; she meticulously maintained records and was an innovator in data collection, tabulation, interpretation and graphical display of descriptive statistics, which she called coxcomb (Joint Commission of resources, 1999).

Sheingold and Hahn (2014) noted that Bismarck style provided universal healthcare for most part of Europe; Chancellor Otto Von Bismarck, fondly known as the father of healthcare in Germany, designed a state-run medical insurance program in 1883 (Sawicki & Bastian, 2008). William Beveridge published the Beveridge Report in 1942 after the second world war, where he described how the healthcare system should be rebuilt and this inspired the vision and formation of the British National Health Service in the year 1948, providing free healthcare at the point of delivery which exists even to this day (Sheingold & A. Hahn, 2014).

During the 20th century, Dr B.C. Roy was a legendary physician, political leader, educationist, philanthropist, social worker and also served as the Chief Minister of West Bengal; he was also rightly called the Maker of Modern West Bengal. After the completion of his MRCP and FRCS, he served as a Professor of Medicine and a Fellow of the American Society of Tropical Medicine and Hygiene, and as the Vice-Chancellor of Calcutta University; he created many institutions including the Indian Institute of Mental Health and The Infectious Disease Hospital which was also the first postgraduate medical college in Kolkata (Kalra, 2011).

DR B.C Roy was instrumental in creating the Indian Medical Association (IMA) in the year 1928 and in making IMA the largest professional organisation within the country; He contributed to the association in many capacities, including being the national president for two terms; The Medical Council of India was his brainchild and despite his hectic political duties as an MLA, Mayor and Chief Minister, he devoted one hour each day to the poor patients and the medical profession (Kalra, 2011).

Leadership in the 20th and 21st century

Formal leadership studies in the western world date back about 100 odd years. After the second world war, many industries started to crop up across the globe and that was when management and leadership concepts started gaining momentum, mainly in the western world.

The leadership that evolved matched the changes that happened in society. In the industrial era, leadership was based on Newtonian principles, organisations worked within defined boundaries and they were functional and predictable; Fredrick Taylor laid down principles for scientific management and through the 1960s business organisations were hierarchical, employees trained on the job and the organisation owned the work of their employees (Porter O'Grady and Melloch, 2011).

As cited by Sheingold & Hahn (2014), in the year 1908, Henry Ford's assembly lines were adapting efficient management systems to increase productivity and reduce wastage; his 'six-sigma lean method' was also adopted by Toyota firm in Japan, the British National Health Service in the UK even though it was meant for the automobile industry as Ford said, "We are charged with discovering the best way of doing everything" (Zarbo and D' Angelo, 2006).

The leadership style in the 20th century mainly involved organising, leading, directing, controlling, informing, parenting, telling, managing, evaluating and was inside-out, top-down, centralised, autocratic, patriarchal and transactional (Strock, 2016) in nature.

In the current world, it is not the organisation but the worker who owns his work; the job descriptions are technical and complex and one needs to be trained to procure jobs; furthermore, the organisation's dependence on the 'worker' has shifted the 'locus of control' from the organisation to the employee, changing the equation of power; the leadership behaviours in the 21st century has a holistic approach. It moved from individual-centred to group-centred, involving spirit and learning, which inspires action and mind (Porter O'Grady and Melloch, 2011).

The leadership behaviour in the 21st century involves enrolling, investing, conflicting, challenging, moderating, facilitating, stretching, and serving as a clearing house, which is based on relationships, outside-in, bottom-up, intuitive, involving soft skills, and is transformational in approach (Strock, 2016).

The internet has become the primary business tool, fibre optics and satellite technology connecting people through seamless networks, miniaturisation, where people, even though mobile, are still connected to everybody and everything, and globalisation has removed boundaries changing the script of our lives; on the whole, in the 20th century, the focus was on performing the correct processes but in the 21st century the focus is on obtaining the right outcomes (Porter O'Grady and Melloch, 2011).

Leadership in Healthcare at Present

As the world stepped out of the 20th century, healthcare across the world faced too many challenges. Working with limited resources, shortage of trained staff, increased regulations, etc. In this century, the tables have turned around; the employee owns his work, his talent and his certified specialisation, and is employed and paid for his specialist work and inputs.

Healthcare in this century yearns for leaders who work not only for their organisations and their employees but at the same time pay importance to the bigger picture (Porter O'Grady and Melloch, 2011). Healthcare in this century also yearns for doctors who not only cater to patients but at the same time pay importance to the all-round performance of the organisation in terms of growth, delivering quality care, and providing overall good patient outcomes, productivity and profits.

In the era of the Internet, mobile phones, digital platforms and artificial intelligence, connecting people far away, including the remote areas that were difficult to reach previously, is now only a button away. The face of healthcare delivery has changed enormously. Globalisation and medical tourism have set our country on the healthcare map.

Are Management and Leadership the Same?

There is one debate that always goes on; are management and leadership one and the same? Not all leaders are managers and not all managers are leaders holds true to the word. Leaders inspire, create a vision, strategize, build a team and help overcome hurdles, concentrating on issues both inside and outside the organisation.

Managers mainly adhere to the processes, work on plans given by their heads and monitor outcomes, performance and work within the organisation.

A leader necessarily need not be a manager. However, a manager needs to possess leadership qualities and skills to perform his role well. Leaders perform much better when they possess excellent managerial skills. It has become imperative for doctors to possess good managerial and leadership skills to work in these times.

Why are leadership qualities important for doctors in today's healthcare setup?

The journey that one embarks on, in the medical field begins the day one sets foot in medical school. The competition, the grasp of the subject, the first steps into clinical postings, dealing with colleagues and mentors, the challenges that medical students face, treating a patient as an intern, through post-graduation or being a specialist consultant, the survival and thriving ability comes with imbibing leadership qualities.

Leadership keenly is not about trying to stand out of the crowd, holding a mike in hand, or getting the best grades; it does not mean that one needs to be a CEO. It is about efficiently handling situations that we come across both on the professional and personal front on a day-to-day basis; it is about working in teams, uplifting one another and achieving the best we can. Failure is never a dead-end. One must remember that failure is an opportunity to retrospect, learn more and get better insight and is a stepping stone for a million opportunities.

There is nothing more thriving than having a healthy set of friends, colleagues and mentors through training, thereafter, at work and in life. Moreover, for those who have not been fortunate, be it having to deal with bureaucracy, bully culture, favouritism, lack of healthy competition, a hostile environment, personal challenges in life or dealing with difficult patients or their kin; one must be able to adapt depending on the situation and circumstances in handling these the best we can. Growth is never easy; life is not a bed of roses, but there are no problems or challenges that do not have solutions or alternative approaches.

In the medical field, informed decisions are made daily; it could be the mode of treatment or the running of the healthcare organisation. One must harness leadership skills to deal with the decisions we make, big or small. Having to deal with challenges and handling teams and various people of different personality types needs tact.

It is vital to be farsighted and think of a solution from various perspectives. For example, while making a treatment choice, choosing to work in a particular organisation, starting a private practice or planning to open your own setup, there are many things to ponder.

There are various options to choose from. One may be comfortable working in a government setup, while the other may opt to work in a nursing home or a corporate; others are happy setting up a small private establishment and another may want to set up a chain of hospitals.

It is essential to be wise in choosing what keeps one satisfied and fulfilled; choose aptly considering expertise, qualifications and the ability to sustain in the culture of the given environment and the resources available. Choose to do what tends to feed personal ambition based on ability. Some prefer not to take any risks, and are pretty satisfied with job security, while few push beyond it and can take it well and there are those who take highly calculated risks. There is nothing right or wrong with any of the choices; what is important is how you can sail your ship.

There are occasions when one may serve too much on their plate, leading to stress and tension causing unpleasant outcomes; this is where teamwork, new approaches and innovation comes into play. Such occasions call for transformational changes, accepting and adapting to change and steadily climbing back up on the positive high of the graph.

A Small Note on Values and Ethics

The minute one steps into the medical field, values and ethics become second skin to most doctors and patients' well-being becomes a priority, so much so that they give up on their personal life and compromise their health and well-being. The noble thoughts and deeds of the medical fraternity are etched within their souls.

Advancements, innovations, corporate culture and involvement of the non-medical players in the healthcare industry, have still kept this nature intact for most doctors, which is phenomenal and has remained despite all the challenges the doctors face on the professional and personal front at the workplace.

Healthcare leaders face many challenging decision-making; be it operational dilemmas in the healthcare organisation, such as allocating budget and revenue generation; or therapeutic decision-making, such as treatment choices. Sometimes, there are grey areas; one has to be wise in making the right decisions that have fair outcomes.

Physicians need to set exemplary grounds in maintaining the moral values of the healthcare organisation within their department and teams, and also maintain great work culture. Good leaders must realise their values and deal with situations and issues that may erupt in the workplace. It may be regarding different treatment options, certain decisions among team members, or it can be healthy competition between colleagues.

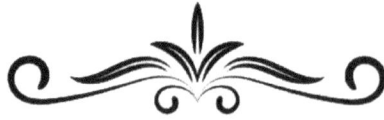

CHAPTER 2

DEFINITION AND APPROACHES TO LEADERSHIP

There are too many definitions of leadership out there, in fact, a very significant number of them. Leadership is a process where the leader motivates and inspires his team in achieving certain aims or objectives.

A leader is one who paints an inspiring vision of the future that is practical and very much achievable, collects a team that possesses the required skillsets, motivates them and manages the delivery of the set goals. A leader deals with any challenges faced by his organisation and team members and is the driving force in keeping his team members on the same page.

Theories of Leadership

The approaches and theories of leadership are borrowed from western countries; the studies and concepts of leadership gained momentum after the second world war.

Because leadership is complex in nature, there are many ways one can approach leadership:

- The Great Man theory
- Trait Theory

- Functional Approach
- Behavioural Theory
- Contingency Theory
- Transactional Leadership Theory
- Transformational Leadership Theories

Other Leadership styles and Leadership theories

- Autocratic Leadership
- Shared Leadership
- Distributed Leadership
- Collaborative Leadership
- Democratic leadership
- Authentic Leadership
- Servant Leadership
- Ethical Leadership

Here are some of the popular theories and styles.

The Great Man Theory (1940s)

The Great Man theory evolved somewhere around the mid-19th century. Thomas Carlyle was one of the first modern writers of leadership and the first one to have ever documented regarding Great Man theory, which implied that only some men are superior to others and these supermen are the ones who quite popularly become our heroes. The Great Man theory assumes that great leaders are born and not created (Madanchian et. al. 2016). They tend to rise time and again when situations arise.

Then, the point to ponder upon is, what made people leaders? Was it to do with traits that they possess or do they 'learn' to evolve as leaders? This slowly led to people wondering about the trait theory.

Trait Theory (1930s-1940s)

The trait theory harbours on the person or an individual rather than the task they perform; an apt example to quote would be Nelson Mandela whose traits included humility, peace-loving nature, bravery, tactical skills, determination, charisma, courage, focus, endurance and forgiving nature to name a few.

Peter Drucker (1954) in his "The Practice of Management" explained that leadership cannot be substituted, created or promoted, nor can it be learnt or taught suggesting that leaders are those with certain particular traits or qualities which make them stand out from the others either by their possession of charisma, integrity, intelligence, confidence, etc. (Northouse 2011).

Common traits that leaders possess is the ability to influence others, the capacity to motivate, having a creative mind, confidence, people skills, courage, being assertive when the need arises, understanding team needs, being adaptable and enthusiastic to take up responsibility.

Stogdill (1948), in his studies, suggested that constitutional and physical factors such as appearance, height, personality and health influence to an extent; being exuberantly self-confident and having higher levels of intelligence that need to be channelised in the right direction and flow, is exceptionally important; emotional stability and being in control of emotions like fear, anger, jealousy, envy, anxiety, etc. is essential.

Good leaders have excellent decision-making skills. They face challenges head-on, are flexible and adapt to circumstances and situations. They also have practical visions and foresight, communicate well with everyone along the echelon and other leaders, as each call for different techniques of communication; they own up to responsibilities and are courageous, trustworthy, showcase empathy and are motivational and not to mention possess skills that are required to be an inspirational role model.

The one flaw of trait theory is that, not all who possess these traits necessarily become leaders. It is also determined by the position they hold at the workplace, which means it depends on the situation.

Functional Approach to Leadership

Adair's (1934), Functional Approach to leadership looks at the functions of leaders rather than the personality of the individual.

The functional leadership theory suggests that leadership depends not only on the leader but the team. The task in question is achieved only when the team members work in harmony and synchrony and is based on steps taken by the team. The popular functional leadership models are John Adair's Action Centred Leadership model and the one by Kouzes and Posner.

Adair's model comprises three components which are the task, team and individual, where the task is the challenge that needs to be carried out by the team who needs to work together to achieve the shared goal and the individual/team member always looks for encouragement and motivation from their colleagues, their leader and the organisation.

Kouzes and Posner (1987), in their book 'The Leadership Challenge' describe 5 sequential behavioural practices:

1. Challenging the process
2. Inspiring a shared vision
3. Enabling others to act
4. Modelling the way
5. Encouraging the heart

Behavioural Theories (1940-1950)

Behavioural leadership is based on imbibing certain behaviours and actions. Also popularly known as the 'style theory,' it enables a person to practice and learn specific behaviours, allowing flexibility in adapting to circumstances that predicts outcomes as a leader. Behavioural theory suggests that certain behaviours differentiate between leaders and non-leaders in a particular given situation (Mullins et al., 2005; Northouse, 2011).

The Ohio State Leadership Studies identified two groups:

Ohio State University conducted studies directed by Shartle (1957) and involved utilising 'The Leader Behaviour Description Questionnaire (LBDQ)' that was formulated by the staff of the Personnel Research Board.

The studies were conducted on members of varied groups such as the military involving the navy and air force, in the field of education involving school principals, teachers, college students and industrial companies to mention a few (Stogdill, 1963). They found two predominant behaviours after analysing the results.

People-oriented leaders: Here, leaders pay attention to the individual needs of clients and employees and focus on mentoring, motivating, listening and showing care and support towards members, hence, improving relations.

Task-oriented leaders: This leadership approach is based on achieving set tasks rather than managing people; it is more structured, operation-based and focuses on outcomes rather than paying attention to employee progress and day-to-day developments.

As cited by Bryman et al., (2011), the task-oriented style helps increase efficiency whereas the relationship-oriented behaviour improves human resources and relations.

Douglas McGregor, a psychologist in the 1960s who put forth the XY theory, suggested two basic approaches in managing people which look at leadership as a behavioural approach.

The X Theory approach assumes people don't like to work and need to be controlled, directed, forced, or punished in achieving organisational goals and further assumes that people preferred to be treated in such ways to avoid any responsibility and preferred security.

Theory Y assumes that people are committed to organisational goals, seek responsibility, use creativity, are intellectual and work comes naturally to them.

The managers who endorse Theory X are often dead-line driven, intolerant, arrogant, not open to suggestions, short-tempered, will not reward, are not participative, and do not involve in team building.

The managers who endorsed Theory X failed to achieve their goals because of the authoritarian management style. Whereas the ones who endorsed Theory Y were more successful because of a more participative nature which relates well to the democratic style of leadership.

Other styles include participative leadership and status-quo leadership, which have a balanced approach, dividing attention between employee progress and increasing company productivity. There are also dictatorial leaders, indifferent leaders, opportunistic leaders (adapt depending on the situation), country club leaders (put employee satisfaction as a top priority), sound leaders and the paternalistic type that come under the behavioural group.

Contingency theory

Contingency theory is based on the fact that there is no single style of leadership that suits all situations. One of the first such models was developed by Fiedler (1958) in his '*Leader Attitudes and Group Effectiveness*' which views leadership from a situational perspective and is based on the style of leadership and the environmental conditions of the particular situation.

His theory states that effective leadership is not only dependent on the style but also based on the situation and conditions that influence it. An individual can be an excellent leader in a certain circumstance but maybe inefficient in another. There are three aspects to consider in the contingency approach: leadership style, the situation and to see who suits best for that particular situation.

Transactional Leadership theory (1970)

Max Weber, a sociologist, first described transactional leadership; further, Bernard M. Bass contributed vastly in the 1980s.

Transactional leaders set clear goals, establish tasks and targets for each team member, motivate, guide employees and hold significant positions within the organisation. For transactional leaders to prove successful, a leader gives rewards to the ones performing well or takes action against those not performing to motivate them to achieve favoured goals.

Leadership is based on a 'give and take' ethos, where the employee performs well and is rewarded and lack of performance is noted and taken to task. A very familiar example is when a cricket team is praised for a win, encouraged and celebrated and a loss criticised and frowned upon with an expectation of a better future performance.

Transformational Leadership (1970-80)

James MacGregor Burns (1978), in his book 'Leadership', was the first to put forward the concept of "transforming leadership". Burns suggested that transforming leadership is a process wherein the heads and followers assist each other in progressing to a higher level of morale and motivation.

Transforming leaders are almost always inspirational and positively influence their teams. They are passionate, grounded, confident, enthusiastic, energetic and give out high positive vibes impressing every colleague and employee by taking care of their needs, boosting their confidence, motivating them, winning their loyalty and inspiring them to achieve extraordinary performance and outcomes.

Transformational leaders have excellent communication skills, are adept in sensing and solving workplace conflicts and are in tune with the needs of the employees. These leaders take responsibility head-on, do not hesitate to take an informed risk, have high emotional intelligence, adapt quickly to situations and have excellent problem-solving skills. Transformational leaders always empower their teammates to become leaders.

Difference between Transformational and Transactional Leadership

Transactional	Transformational
Caretaker/Mothering approach	Committed approach / Positive influential approach
Barter system approach, award/ punishment approach	Vision-inspired goals/Inspiring employees to strive
Concentrates on task to be achieved	Concentrates on effects and overall growth
Uses rewards/punishment	Empowers others
No shared values	Long term vision
Management oriented tasks	Works on common values
Works with existing culture of the organisation	Strives to change the existing culture for the better of the organisation
Focus on maintaining status quo	Focus is on progression, growth and looking forward

Collaborative Leadership

Al Sawai (2013) suggests that collaborative leaders are very proficient in communicating with their colleagues, employees and with everyone within and outside the organization; this type of leadership involves collaboration and understanding the situation, the goals that need to be achieved, being aware of the negatives and keeping a tab on available manpower and resources that is required; collaborative leaders facilitate organisations and their teams in making informed choices; this type of leadership encourages communication between employees and multiple stakeholders while sharing experiences and knowledge brings out better ideas and innovations that can effectively be utilised to achieve desired goals.

Collaborative leaders bring teams together, earn trust, collaborate work, encourage communication through various means, encourage brainstorming sessions, manage conflicts well and are innovative, hold multiple skill sets, boost staff morale and encourage risk-taking to achieve certain tasks without having to worry about job security. Collaborative leaders are also proficient in managing change, which is constant in the healthcare industry.

Shared Leadership

Practical life experiences and several studies show that most qualified healthcare professionals do not take well to authoritarian leadership. The focus on leadership needs to be towards developing collaborative relationships by distributing workload and task delegation that act as the basis for a shared leadership model within healthcare organizations (Al Sawai 2013).

Shared leadership works well at the team level, say consultants within a particular department. This concept would empower the team members, introduce mutual respect, build confidence and provide a healthy work environment. But it is common to come across failure in establishing this sort of leadership when there is unhealthy competition, poor team ethos, lack of taking responsibility or when the workload is heavy and unequally distributed among its members. Efficient teamwork is the key to the shared-leadership approach, focusing mainly on recognizing team values and efficiency to improve practice.

Distributed Leadership

Distributed leadership is more about increasing the capacity of leadership within the organization where the leads have the ability, competence and autonomy to get the work done at their levels; This type of leadership works towards creating an atmosphere where staff can enhance each other's strengths and offset their weaknesses, with leadership distributed throughout the organization (Al-Sawai, 2013).

As cited by Al-Sawai (2013), distributed leadership calls for four aspects (Garman et. al., 2011) which are:

- Sense-making: the ability to interpret the constantly evolving changes within the business environment and translate these changes to all facets of the organisation.
- Relating: trust building, ability to grow networks of supportive trustworthy people.
- Visioning: creating realistic and compelling visions for the future
- Inventing: developing new ways of approaching tasks and problems

Emotional Intelligence (EQ)

As cited by Chaidi & Drigas (2022), Goleman, in the late 1990s, suggested that five critical competencies make up emotional intelligence: self-awareness (knowing own strengths and weaknesses), self-regulation (managing emotions well), social skills (ability to direct people by interacting well), empathy (considering peoples feeling while interacting) and motivation (being driven to achieve). Much has been written about EQ in business research and social sciences. The concept of EQ does lag in the healthcare industry and may be beneficial, especially when considering nurse leadership.

People skills are very much necessary to have successful careers. Several leaders or many talented people, despite having great skill sets, high IQ and knowledge, still fail because they lack emotional intelligence.

One of the main aims while writing this book was, for doctors to be able to recognize their strengths and work on their weaknesses. Self-awareness makes one identify their weaknesses and strengths. People with high EQ are considerate, reflect on their actions and work on their flaws. It is well documented now that people with successful careers, score higher on their EQ and the predictability of successful careers are based more on high EQ than high IQ.

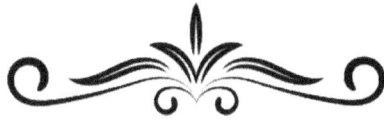

CHAPTER 3

LEADERSHIP STYLES IN HEALTHCARE

*E*very individual is different, every situation is different, and various leadership types or styles can be adopted in healthcare. Healthcare is an ever-evolving arena where the only thing constant is 'change.'

Global and Indian healthcare is growing in costs, clinical advancements, innovation and technology. One has to consider balancing the administrative aspects, managing clinical teams and working within the allocated budget.

When it comes to healthcare leadership, one needs to have a defined vision, have the charisma to influence teams, be a great listener, be open to positive criticism, embrace innovation and advanced technologies, encourage best practices, value ethics and place patients' well-being as a priority.

One can argue whether transactional leadership is better or transformational approach is better, but healthcare professionals can use both styles depending on the situation and circumstance. Achieving targets, progress, productivity and growth are only possible when quality patient-centred care is delivered. This calls for healthcare professionals and managers to have a complete view of the situation while making decisions.

The charisma of an individual plays a vital role in influencing teams; being motivational, sensitive, observant and being able to connect with the team and the task at hand almost always have positive outcomes.

As we advance, new leadership concepts and names are being introduced and more contemporary styles are being expressed when it comes to leadership, but whichever approach is adopted, quality of care delivered to a patient is one of the main criteria in achieving all round success.

'Servant leadership' also has worked well in the healthcare arena, where the central philosophy of the leader is to serve. Robert K. Greenleaf (1970) said, "The leader-first and the servant-first are two extreme types. Between them are shading and blends that are a part of the infinite variety of human nature." He further says, "The difference manifests itself in the care taken by the servant-first to make sure that other people's highest priority is being served. The best test and difficult to administer is: do those served become healthier, wiser, freer, more autonomous, more likely themselves to become servants?" A servant leader is an empath, healer, aware of feelings, weaknesses and strengths, a good listener, uses persuasion, has foresight, conceptualisation, stewardship and uses the available resources well.

Collaborative leadership works well at the top management level, while shared leadership works better at team levels. CEOs, medical directors, medical administrators, nurse managers, etc., hold important positions, giving them the authority to formally lead. However, leading is just not about 'the role or position' as there have been numerous examples of ineffective leads who have held important positions and those that have been exceptionally great leaders and did not have a significant post.

Adaptive leadership and leadership beyond boundaries and authority have increased significantly in organisations adopting a transformational approach.

Some leaders adopt an autocratic leadership style; this style does not work when there are multiple stakeholders involved and can be disastrous for the organisation. Though authoritarian leadership faces a lot of criticism, sometimes, it may be the only way forward. More so when autocratic leadership is adopted by an individual with a transformational streak, especially while making decisions in an emergency or while making decisions critical in nature, it can be vital and productive. If an individual owns the organisation and they aim to steer the direction of their organisation towards a desired set of goals, autocratic leadership is beneficial; during organisational unrest and a transformational change process, autocratic leadership style comes in very handy.

Democratic and laissez fare styles are good styles to adopt in the healthcare industry that empowers clinical professionals to make their departmental decisions; nurses being empowered and managers at floor levels given lead roles, after being educated and sensitised to the importance of quality patient care, have productive outcomes.

Network-based approach has been gaining importance, both within and outside the healthcare arena. In the Indian healthcare system, the government, policymakers, private and public sectors, individual health organisations—small or large, be it charity or NGO supported, rural/ urban—need to work in unison towards a shared purpose and envision giving patient-centred quality healthcare.

During the work process, informal relationships are formed through shared work that improves communication between colleagues within and outside the organisation. This creates a network that facilitates required resources, support, information and word-by-mouth marketing, which enhances and influences the progress of an organisation or an individual's career path. Hence, networking becomes essential.

At the end of it, different situations and circumstances call for different approaches and tact; healthcare leaders and clinicians need to be confident; informed, have all the required skills and knowledge, keep up to date with the trends in the industry and be up-to-date with innovations and work towards change.

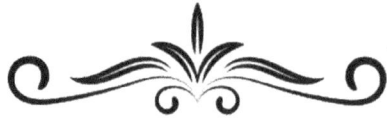

CHAPTER 4

CONFLICT MANAGEMENT AND COMMUNICATION

Conflict Management and Leadership

Conflicts are not uncommon at a workplace, home or in personal life-related situations. Mastering conflict management is an essential life skill to prevent adverse impacts on oneself and those involved while attaining positive outcomes against all odds.

A new change to a situation or a disagreement can lead to a lot of distress, which can be avoided with good conflict management strategies.

Within an organisation, conflicts can arise due to selfish behaviours, lack of communication, when stakeholders are not on the same page, when there is a discrepancy between the expectation and needs of the stakeholders and employees, clashes in perceptions and personal values, competition for power and top management roles; or for that matter, it is not uncommon to see conflicts between two consultants in the same department over various issues.

Conflict within healthcare organisations, between the management and the front-line staff, between different teams, conflict of ideas between stakeholders, between the non-medical and the clinical teams, etc., can give rise to gaps and have an impact on the outcomes in quality care, the services and set goals. Conflicts arise time and again and it is vital to know how to deal with them.

Stages of Conflict

Latent stage – Where the team is not aware of the conflict.

Perceived stage – Where the team senses the conflict.

Felt stage – Involves a lot of tension and stress.

Manifest stage – Facing the conflict; this is the noticeable state.

Aftermath – Outcome

Healthcare leaders need to employ strategies to manage conflict at all stages, creating positive outcomes for everyone involved. Various techniques such as compromise, collaboration, negotiation, facilitating communication, mediation, seeking consensus, bargaining, competition, avoidance, etc., can be employed to facilitate the resolution of conflict.

Solving a conflict through compromise requires cooperation and assertiveness from the groups involved, while disputes dealt by accommodating requires more cooperation from parties involved.

Trying to resolve conflict by avoidance is another ball game; it needs tact but, at the same time, can give rise to more challenges. The conflict can keep cropping up time and again and can snowball into a bigger issue, which also causes a lot of hurt and dissatisfaction. Solving conflicts by avoidance is best avoided.

Competing or conflict management by force is not very popular and best avoided in most situations. But when conflicts arise when a leader needs to bring about change, or when it is a pressing issue, competing conflict management skills come in handy; but other methods should be pondered upon before utilising this approach.

A collaborative approach to conflict management is beneficial for all those concerned and benefits everyone involved; this sort of resolving conflict is best for equal stakeholders and those with equal power vested in them.

Conflicts often give rise to resentment, pain, hurt, heartbreak, increased stress, anxiety and depression; it can result in low self-esteem, low staff morale, frustration and aggression.

The first step in dealing with a conflict is to acknowledge an issue that needs resolving. It is essential to gather detailed information from all the parties involved. Set specific goals, strategies and rules to abide by while attentively listening and avoiding emotional outbursts and anger as they are not permanent solutions; they will need addressing at some point. Using appropriate strategies and skilled conflict management techniques to resolve the issue always comes in handy.

Communication — An Integral Part of Leadership

The most happening buzzword, not only in healthcare but every other field, is 'communication'. Communication is the crux of any relationship or negotiation. A good leader is expressive, a good communicator and a good listener. Communication plays a vital role— be it communicating with patients, their relatives, teams, the hospital management or other non-medical staff in the hospital. Lack of communication can lead to poor patient care and hamper the hospital's delivery of services, goals and achievements.

A leader needs to be inclusive and hear out the employees, teams and non-medical staff. Many hospital staff cites a lack of communication or inability to approach their leads, resulting in poor quality of services. Good communication should be engraved within the culture of the organisation. Lack of communication between stakeholders, from heads to employees or within teams, leads to bad outcomes and negatively impacts employees' morale.

Transformational leaders with excellent communication skills, who engage well with all the employees always perform better and achieve favourable outcomes. Trust, good listening skills, proper duty hand-overs and avoiding miscommunication play a vital role in departmental and inter-departmental functioning, leading to good quality care.

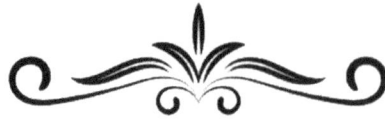

CHAPTER 5

ORGANISATIONAL CULTURE

*O*rganisational culture gained attention since the 1980s. In straightforward terms, organisational culture is what the organisation is. It is how things are done in an organisation; they are the values, norms and beliefs that all members share. Culture is the soul that determines how a group of people behave. Culture is commonly shared beliefs that, in turn, shape the behaviours of individuals.

Why is it important to understand culture? It is because culture and leadership are two sides of the same coin and one can only be understood with the other (Schien, 1995). It is equally important to know that within these cultures bask subcultures, giving rise to complexities. Organisations have subcultures based on similar occupations, specialities, skill-sets and shared histories.

Mintzberg et al. (2009) profess that the culture school is the mirror image of power school, implying that culture and power are entwined. Culture depends significantly on the driving force meaning—those holding influential positions within the organisation. The cultures and subcultures influence the organisation's functions and contribute to strategic capabilities. Schein (1992) describes culture in three deep levels—the first level as artefacts, what one sees, hears and feels as one enters a particular atmosphere; level two, the espoused principles, values, ethics and vision; level three, underlying assumptions, which are taken for granted beliefs.

Organisational Culture in Healthcare

In today's world, healthcare has become global and industrialised, attracting investors from varied backgrounds, involving mergers, joint ventures and acquisitions requiring people to work between cross cultures. India has a dominant private healthcare sector. It is vital for every individual in the healthcare profession, clinical and non-clinical, to develop awareness and nurture healthy work cultures and realise that apart from organisational goals, a safe work environment and compassionate patient-centred care should be the shared vision of every organisation, and that obtaining competitive advantage should be through fair means.

There are few studies conducted on how culture in healthcare influences performance. Still, we must recognise that there is enough evidence that good work cultures positively impact performance in studies conducted in the other industrial sectors.

As healthcare evolved in our country, work culture has simultaneously evolved. A couple of decades ago, general physicians played a vital role in providing healthcare; the doctors were almost like extended family members. Things have changed; more and more people are opting for specialist care and many patients prefer private or corporate health establishments, especially in urban areas. The government has devised various schemes to make healthcare affordable to many. As healthcare saw transition, culture saw changes at all levels, from artefacts to assumptions, vision and beliefs. There is one thing that has remained firmly rooted and remains unshakable: the dedication and the way our doctors provide clinical care to their patients despite all challenges and transitional changes they face in their place of work.

A healthy work atmosphere in hospitals, say between the leader and the employees, clinical and non-clinical teams create a positive environment with favourable outcomes. Hierarchy has been quite traditional when it comes to healthcare; bureaucracy is rampant at all levels, making things more complex and causing much unhappiness amongst caregivers. Those from non-healthcare backgrounds are far removed from 'healthcare' and it is likely that they make decisions that can hamper the quality-of-care delivery. It is vital to have people with trained backgrounds who are sensitive and understand that healthcare is an arena where the quality of care cannot be compromised.

Organisational Culture and Leadership

Culture drives the way we behave within and outside the organisation. Various cultures influence us; be it the culture at home, within the society where we obtained our education, our professional circles, etc., cultures are a part of us and influence us. As and when situations arise, we take on roles of leaders, which will not only impress upon the present culture but gives rise to new cultural dimensions.

If an entrepreneur opens a new organisation, he will create visions, norms, and behaviours that will define the type of leadership within that organisation. Say, if an autocrat created a successful organisation, the employees would see that leadership as the right way. On the other hand, if a democratic leader creates a successful organisation, the employees believe that it is indeed the correct way. The whole confusion, then, of defining the 'right type' of leadership has been challenging and many organisations have had their own approach and done exceptionally well (Schien, 1995).

If the organisation had a new leader or CEO, there would be a few possibilities. The leader would have to choose from specific options, either destroy the existing culture, fight the current culture, give into the existing culture or evolve the existing culture.

This brings us to realise that change is constant, and for many leaders, this would be a preferred option, which is to increase effectiveness, this is called "culture change" (Schien, 1995), and change calls for brilliant leaders and managers along the echelon.

In a hospital scenario, for example, a new HOD, consultant, or clinician took over a department and thought that things could be more efficient, which would call for decisions to be made. The task would involve coordinating, teamwork, allocating responsibilities, empowering team members, having shared leadership goals, teaching, and so much more, which requires leadership skills.

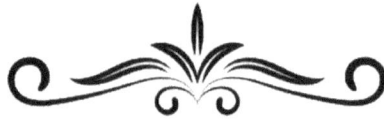

CHAPTER 6

CHANGE MANAGEMENT

*A*t the beginning of the 20th century, when management evolved as a subject, academics and practitioners gave importance to change management. Change management gained more prominence after the second world war, during which complex organisations emerged worldwide. Much work has been done in the area of change in the last eighty-odd years.

Ginter et al. (2013), acknowledge evolutionary changes came about in the healthcare industry in the 1980s. Change is a process rather than an event and is dependent on decisions made by the members rather than the organisation per say. It is a personal experience for the ones involved and is a gradual process of growth and skills.

Many issues need attention in the healthcare industry and applying concepts that evolved several years ago can make a huge difference. Healthcare has been growing at a great pace, but more recently, evolutionary changes have come about in the healthcare industry.

There is always resistance to change because the ones involved feel they will suffer the consequences of change. Change requires erasing old habits of work patterns.

Working towards change is a calculated risk that has to be taken. And how smoothly this process occurs depends on the ones leading the change process.

With change, comes various insecurities and fears. To name a few, employees may face the fear of loss of job and its consequences for them, fear of financial burdens, there is lack of confidence, unrest, non-acceptance, say of a certain process or new strategy and there is resistance to change. On the other hand, the stakeholders have their own set of risks involved. It is not uncommon to come across fear, frustration, anger, hopelessness, constant questioning, complaints, quitting work, absenteeism, and conflicts among employees. There are various approaches to change. Planned change is a deliberate act involving conscious decision-making and reasoning while emergent change unfolds unplanned and spontaneously.

There is also episodic and continuous change; according to Weick and Quinn (1999), change can be episodic, i.e. intentional, infrequent and discontinuous, while continuous change is ongoing, where people adapt continuously and work towards evolving and growing. It is quite interesting to note that episodic change caters to transactional goals while continuous change caters to transformational goals.

Ackerman's (1997), described three kinds of change:

Developmental Change – Involves working with the existing issues within the organisation and can be planned or emergent.

Transactional Change – Works towards achieving a desired goal from the currently existing state and can be planned, emergent or radical.

Transformational Change – Works towards a shift in beliefs and assumptions i.e. culture, strategy, bringing about changes in processes and structures in achieving significant milestones from the existing stage. Transformational change can be radical in nature and can drift into a developmental mode that is continuously working towards growing, improving and adapting.

Working towards change in the organisation means working with change in behaviours and the way people approach to new changes. Most of the time, employees tend to find themselves in a 'comfort zone' where they feel a sense of belonging, familiar, unthreatened, and there is a sense of predictability in the work patterns. It is important for leaders to nudge their staff into a 'discomfort zone' which is a place where people are uncertain, willing to adapt to change and change process (NHS England). There is something called the 'panic zone'. A good leader will do everything to prevent his staff from getting into the panic zone, where people freeze, which is where all the feelings of dissatisfaction, anger, stress, feelings of inferiority build up and people will not adapt or even consider working towards change. People will not learn to adapt to change when in the 'panic zone'.

As Kevin Cashman (2014) phrases it, *"Being 'comfortable with discomfort' activates the heart of transformation."* The 'panic zone' can be avoided when leaders cushion their employees, give them enough time to cope with the situation and encourage internal communication within the organisation. People need to feel safe, which calls for great leadership skills. Leadership that facilitates change involves prioritising work, granting rewards, allowing employees to express their worries and grief, acknowledging things that did not go right, involving training, forming a support group, reassuring, providing employees with a compelling vision to work towards, which makes the change process much more acceptable and smooth.

Decision-making

Decision-making, meaning choosing a course of action from the alternatives available in today's complex and dynamic health setup can be quite challenging (Ozcan A.,2009); due to the complexity involved in the problems being faced, the managers have a huge task at hand. However, these decisions might have been based on unspoken or unconscious assumptions related to the organisation, its future and the environment

(Mintzberg, 1989). Decision implementation involves behavioural skills such as influence and leadership; accurate identification of the problem is a very significant part of the process; a problem that is defined well is probably half the solution found (Ozcan A.,2009); often the managers tend to focus on the symptoms of the problem rather than focussing on the root causes that results in the problems re-surfacing over and over again (Ozcan A., 2009).

Use of Tools

Various tools are used in change management; no single tool, model or method will work well with all problems or situations. It strongly depends on the complexity of the situation, the interdependence and fragmentation within the organisation; application of the strategic models and tools can be used for various purposes, either to make strategies, bring about organisational changes or to analyse a particular problem arising within or outside the organisation (Iles and Sutherland, 2001).

Below is an example of Kotter's eight steps for change management:

Kotter's eight steps of change management (2002)

1. Create a sense of urgency
   - Help make employees realise the importance and need for change
   - Identify opportunities and crises at hand
2. Build a guiding coalition
   - Collect a group with the needed skills and power to lead the change process
   - Encourage teamwork
3. Form a strategic vision
   - Sketch visions to direct change and strategies to achieve those visions.
4. Communicate the vision
   - Utilise mechanisms, involve many for the communication of vision
   - Empower new behaviours

5. Enable action by uprooting barriers
   - Uproot barriers and obstacles to change
   - Act beyond non-traditional ideas and actions
   - Encourage risk-taking
   - Appreciate, reward and recognise new achievements
6. Generate short-term wins
   - Create achievements through small milestones
   - Create and set aims that are achievable
   - Start new after completing the current phases
7. Sustain acceleration
   - Be determined and persistent
   - Consolidatie improvements and work towards more change
8. Institutionalise change
   - Weave the change into the 'culture'
   - Ensuring succession and leadership development
   - Articulating connection between the newly acquired behaviour and success

Kotter (2002) gave probable reasons as to why the change process fails and that includes the complexity involved, lack of efficient coalition, lack of clear visions, barriers to the achievable visions, lack of communication to share the vision, declaring victory prematurely and importantly, the failure to engrave the 'change' in the existing culture.

There are many tools, frameworks, models and techniques to choose from, like the SWOT Analysis that helps assess why we need the change. SWOT and PEST analysis are used often as strategic assessment tools; Force Field Analysis is a popular analysing/planning tool (Iles and Sutherland, 2001). There are various other tools to consider, like The McKinsey 7-S change management model, Bridges' transition change management model, PDSA cycle, Ackerman and Anderson's 9-stage model and Kubler-Ross's 5-stage change management model to name a few.

Kurt Lewin (1952), fondly called the funder of modern social psychology, created the 3-step change management model and the Force Field Theory.

Lewin's three-stage model constitutes three stages of the change process, which are unfreezing, the change process itself and the freezing stage.

Lewin's three-stage model -

Freeze - Prepare, communicate, and provide clarity.

Change process/Transition – The process of moving towards change.

Refreeze – Stabilizing new norms and behaviours.

Lewin's Force Field Analysis, explains how the change process works by understanding the driving and restraining forces that facilitate the change. It is important to diagnose the driving and restraining forces. On one hand, there are the driving forces, for example, poor patient feedback, low profits, and decreased employee satisfaction. On the other hand, are the restraining forces like staff shortage, growing competition, and staff who insecure about newer technology. While the driving force navigates the organisation towards desired change, the restraining forces cause resistance. According to Kurt Lewin, stability is achieved when both the above-described forces reach equilibrium, i.e. which are equal strength from either direction.

In conclusion, public or private healthcare organisations need to work towards embracing continuous emergent change. This shift depends on the government, corporate healthcare sector, healthcare professionals and managers at all levels of the echelon. Handling change in a complex environment with conflicting objectives, multiple stakeholders, significant constraints and the amalgamation of various cultures and subcultures is challenging. Different tools are available and managers must be careful in choosing a tool best suited for that particular situation.

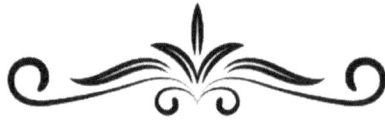

CHAPTER 7

LEADERSHIP, PSYCHOLOGY AND TRANSFERENCE

$\mathcal{P}$eople are in awe of the ones that stand apart from the rest. Is it any particular trait that they showcase? Are they born leaders, or does genetics matter? Some individuals are born with a golden spoon, everything ready on a platter; does that make them good leaders? Does the environment, opportunity or education matter? Do autocratic leadership or narcissistic traits fetch better results or fail to achieve desired goals?

It is safe to say that even if an individual has all the traits or was a born leader, opportunity, intelligence, education, training, and various external factors play a vital role in shaping a leader. As discussed earlier, leadership is also situational. Task-oriented or relationship-oriented leadership, each work well depending on the situation. Transactional leadership helps one meet the desired task, whereas transformational leadership helps one achieve the desired goals. Hence, it is essential to adopt to various styles depending on the situation.

Autocratic leadership is rampant, especially in small healthcare set-ups with very few employees but may help jobs get done quickly. Still, it is not uncommon to see autocratic leaders who run medium - large organisations. Autocratic leadership is not the right approach to achieving desired goals, especially in medium-large organisations with multiple stakeholders. The authoritarian leadership style probably works when it's a do-or-die situation where things must be acted upon quickly.

Autocratic leaders are far removed from the concerns or opinions of the employees and the challenges they face, and there is lack of communication. The autocrat dictates the task that needs to be carried out with no questions asked, leading to dissatisfaction among staff resulting in a lack of morale among employees.

As cited by (Kets de Vries & Miller, 1984), Freud states, "The leader himself need love no one else, he may be of a masterful nature, absolutely narcissistic, self-confident and independent" (1921). He also described narcissistic libidinal personality where an individual's main focus is self-preservation; this individual is independent and difficult to intimidate. Freud (1931) believed that such people are suited to impress others and are ideological or moral bastions and true leaders (Kets de Vries & Miller, 1984).

Narcissism is believed to be a driving force behind the want to obtain the leadership position; those with strong narcissistic personalities are quite willing to take strenuous steps to achieve power; not long ago, narcissistic personality came under critical scrutiny; DSM III listed a number of large criteria to describe narcissistic personality disorders (Kets de Vries & Miller, 1984). In DSM-5, Narcissistic Personality Disorders (NPD), is described as the need for admiration, grandiosity, and lack of empathy and is classified under the dimensional model of "Personality Disorders" presenting with difficulty in maintaining relationships and work (Mitra & Fluyau, 2023).

It must be noted though, that characteristics of narcissism occur with different degrees of intensity. A certain amount of narcissism is needed to function effectively and most of us show signs of narcissistic behaviour (Kets de Vries & Miller, 1984). Those that possess limited tendencies contribute greatly to society; those gravitating towards the extremes head towards pejorative reputations showing rigidity, resistance, narrowness and can have crucial and dramatic implications (Kets de Vries & Miller, 1984).

As Kets de Vries and Miller (1984), put forth, "Leadership can be pathologically destructive or most inspiring."

The narcissistic trait of a leader who lacks empathy, understanding, shows resistance to suggestions, has a critiquing nature, and their thirst to be famous often leads to dissatisfaction, and such leaders break rather than make an organisation.

Some leaders resign or are forced to step down for having failed to achieve the desired vision or have failed to gain love and respect from their stakeholders, colleagues and employees due to their greed for power, position and financial gains. There is dissatisfaction amongst stakeholders due to autocratic or narcissistic behaviour. Such leaders sink the organisation. When one reaches that position and power, it is easy to be obsessed with it but one must stay grounded.

It has been observed that a good leader keeps his employees inspired, happy and keeps his communication doors open at all levels within the organisation. Such organisations perform really well, have a great work culture and good employee satisfaction.

Psychology and leadership have a deep-seated connection, be it the qualities and the influences that shape a leader; their relationships, interaction or influence with the employees and teams; or, for that matter, the way they influence the minds of their teams and the ones they interact with.

What brings employee satisfaction? One is job security, another is the salary. But is that enough to retain staff? Probably not, unless the individual is pressed to compromise. What retains the employees apart from the job and financial security includes the culture within the organisation, the relations and positive interactions they develop with their colleagues, and having a leader who gives attention to detail, is approachable, has empathy and listens to everyone working in his organisation, from his medical to non-medical teams, and the kind of bonds he shares with his stakeholders that results in a positive environment and a great work culture. Employees crave appreciation and praise; it is worth remembering that a small praise goes a long way.

Knowledge of psychology comes in handy when one has to interact with their patients and their families or deal with difficult patients and their families.

Negotiation is another ball game altogether. Knowing or understanding the psychology of the parties involved has its advantages. It may help to understand the pressures, limitations, intent and loyalty of the parties involved and help find strategies that have mutual benefits that bring about more productivity. It also helps when one interacts with people who may try to take advantage of them in a dignified manner through effective EQ-based communication.

What has come to my knowledge is that many things resolve without conflicts, be it something that involves top-level decision-making with high stakes or something as simple as declining a small job of an applicant who has come with hopes and dreams in their eyes. Most things resolve with effective communication and the use of EQ.

For example, one wants to decline a person who has applied for work in the organisation, or it is an in-house consultant that has approached the management with a strategic plan to help the organisation, or some other party that has come to negotiate a business deal, or there is a conflict between colleagues; decline or resolve using EQ depending on the situation because with the knowledge, power, education, should also come empathy, humanness and being humble. Staying grounded takes a leader or a non-leader a long way. There is a certain way to communicate it to an individual for whom being treated in a rude manner can derail their morale, dwindle their confidence, cause hurt, anger, more out of sadness, cause depression and can impact their prospects and have repercussions for years to come in their life. This kind of rude behaviour also reflects the culture within the organisation, especially when it comes from stakeholders and important people in the organisation.

It is not only necessary to take care of what happens within your organisation but outside of it as well; it can be a vendor, a medical representative, someone who has come to negotiate a business or a job applicant; or for that matter while breaking news to an existing employee who has so passionately served the organisation for years, that their services are no longer needed. It is imperative that when they walk out of the door whatever the outcome, be it positive or negative, should do so with a praise and respect of how a process was handled and that calls for high EQ and excellent leadership skills at different strata in the organisation, be it the CEO, marketing head, HR or anyone with responsible positions.

There is no limit to having knowledge about how we humans interact. The knowledge of psychology comes in handy in marketing exercises to impress upon the customers and the clients or to impress parties while handling major mergers.

Transference is a common occurrence in the workplace. Sigmund Freud (1912) believed that transference roots from childhood experiences, where subconsciously, elders such as parents become knights in shining armour who protect them from their fears and provide them with a safe haven; on becoming adults, we tend to transfer this sort of attachments to individuals that provide a sense of security or tame insecurities and fears.

Transference is a phenomenon where an individual directs their feelings or aspirations for one person to another. It is not uncommon for an employee to relate their boss as someone important in their life, say a father or a motherly figure or a brother or a loved one.

Though it is believed that transference occurs most commonly in therapeutic settings with patients undergoing psychological therapy where they subconsciously start to see their therapist as someone important in their life such as a parent, sibling or other, it is as common at workplace. There can also be something called nonfamilial transference.

In fact, transference can very much happen outside of therapeutic settings or workplace, to anyone anywhere, anytime, with people we encounter in day-to-day happenings of life and is believed to stem from early life experiences.

There is also countertransference which binds the leader to his followers and explains his leadership behaviour and determines their interaction and acceptance of each other as leader and followers.

Leaders need to use the power of transference in a positive manner. Using it positively can enhance good organisational outcomes. Transference can sometimes cause negative repercussions; for example, a follower may relate his leader with someone whom he previously has had a bad experience with, and subconsciously behaves rebelliously with his present boss.

There is a possibility of an employee having multiple transferences with different individuals within the organisation, be it with the leads or colleagues. It is not uncommon for employees who are basking in their boss's praises to suddenly lose their morale when the boss has been busy making high stake decisions and is unable to give the employee regular attention.

Countertransference can also be an issue where the leader projects their previous experiences onto the employee. There is a possibility that the leader can start believing this illusion that the love the employee has for them is true and look at the employee as a daughter, son, grandchild, sibling, or other, which can result in favouritism, favoured opportunities and special allowances that may backfire if this employee is not cut out for that role or task at hand and can lead to non-productive or disastrous outcomes.

It can also happen that countertransference can impact the employee negatively if the boss subconsciously relates to an employee as a non-productive ex-employee or someone they have not got along with in the past. It can hinder the interaction with the current employee so much that it can destroy the prospects of this particular employee.

In conclusion, it is essential for leaders to be able to recognise normal conscious behaviours from subconsciously directed behaviours and to be able to handle both situations.

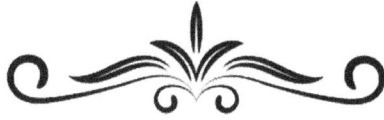

CHAPTER 8

THE LEADERSHIP FRAMEWORK

*M*any countries have a national healthcare leadership framework that blankets all healthcare workers, irrespective of their roles. Having a leadership framework engraves leadership values and ethos into every healthcare worker in the system, both in public and private sectors. This, in turn, builds a healthy work culture within the healthcare system.

A leadership framework helps devise a successful team, enhance their potential, motivate and strategise the road map to success, working towards the desired purpose.

Dhanvantri Framework

The "Dhanvantri Framework" was devised by me after having worked in the industry, having observed and understood the system. This framework, for all practical purposes, is applicable from the grass root level to corporates to government healthcare establishments. The framework has eight components. This framework has been constructed considering both the public and private sectors and can be applicable across both.

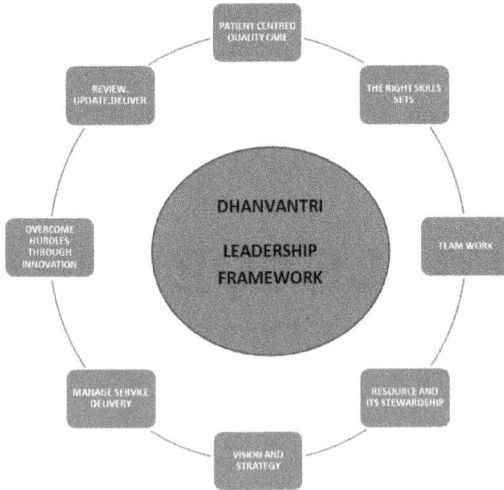

Copy rights reserved Dr Pallavi Hoskote (2023)

1. Patient-centred quality care

The prime goal of healthcare organisations and every individual who works in the healthcare sector, despite the role, should revolve around patient-centred quality care.

2. The right skill sets

It is essential to have the right education, practical knowledge and required skillsets, to achieve the shared purpose. Continuous learning and being up-to-date with new innovations to deliver standard quality care is essential.

Bringing together the right skillsets or team building to achieve the shared purpose is an extremely important aspect. Having the right team is half the battle won. It is essentially important to take on board the right team, and if need be to get the ones that don't contribute off it, after having given all the support and opportunitiy.

3. Teamwork

Teamwork is vital in achieving the set goals of providing quality care; be it one single team of a small healthcare set-up, multiple teams working in synchrony, be it at the hospital level, between large units or departments, or be it at the state level or between networks at the national level, appropriate teams, working in harmony, encouraging and supporting each other becomes essential to achieve the shared purpose.

4. Resource and Resource stewardship

Various resources are essential to provide quality care, such as finance, human resources, equipment, etc. Resources need to be managed well, be it working within a small or large budget, mindfully utilising the funds is necessary. Not only the finances but the workforce and logistics, connecting the dots innovatively and bringing all components together must be done wisely.

5. Vision and strategy

Anything to be achieved always starts with a vision. Here, we are looking at delivering the best quality care to our patients. Appropriate strategies are essential. Having a bird's eye view, identifying drawbacks, gaps and how they can be tackled is crucial. It is always important to have backup strategic plans ready to achieve the purpose just in case bottleneck issues arise.

It is essential to revisit the vision and strategies in place and review them from time to time to know what we are working towards, especially in healthcare, where change is constant, the modes of achieving this shared purpose change with innovations.

6. Managing service delivery

Managing the services is an important aspect as the outcomes depend on it. From making sure good care is being provided, handling hurdles, managing the smooth functioning of the organisation and most importantly, tactful management of the staff and resources rests upon a proficient management team.

7. Overcome hurdles through innovation

As we discussed, change is constant and challenges keep cropping up. Making service delivery flawless with a pleasant experience and reaching out to service users is no straightforward task.

Barriers need to be overcome through innovations. Be it using different modes of service delivery by use of new technologies, advancements, or just the right kind of strategy to reach the customers sums up innovation. Innovations can mean anything from more recent technology, newer devices, equipment, advanced techniques or treatments in the medical field or advanced procedures that enhance safety and better patient outcomes.

Innovation is a man-made creation that the human race is proud of but can backfire if not used rightly. For example, incidents and insecurities can arise in healthcare due to patient information data breaches, issues related to confidentiality and privacy, missing out on the right diagnosis for having been unable to see the patient face to face or misinformation through platforms. It is essential to use it with an evidence-based approach under the legal framework.

8. Review, Update and Deliver

It is essential to have regular reviews and audits of the processes and services. Audit the quality of care being provided and take feedback from the employees, patients and their families seriously and act on it, working on strategies to overcome any breaches or flaws. It is essential to be updated with newer advancements and continue to provide the best care services within given resources and time.

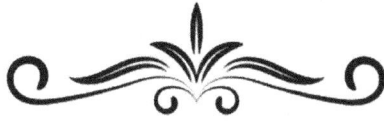

CHAPTER 9

WORKING TOWARDS CHANGE

$\mathcal{P}$orter and Mc Laughlin (2006) express that, many arguments have taken place about the leadership context, comparing it to the weather, discussed only superficially and noticed only at certain times. Tremendous change has occurred as to how context shapes leadership roles.

As cited in Hartley & Bennington (2010), Burns wrote, "Leadership is one of the most observed and least understood phenomena on earth."

The healthcare sector is a highly complex environment, enfolding different departments, nonlinear communication and interactions, varied professional groups, various specialities and having to work with constraints such as budget, demography, politics, multidirectional goals, intricate subcultures and cultural webs, conflicting visions, and healthcare thrives in complexity.

The challenges healthcare leaders face is the diversity within organisations whether it be public or private. Healthcare leaders need to encourage members towards shared goals, utilise resources to design and manage within defined constraints and adopt new changes within the healthcare domain.

Healthcare bills are revised every few years bringing changes within many facets of the healthcare sector throughout the world. There are always tremendous changes in political, social, economic, technological and ecological aspects that impact healthcare delivery.

Working with constraints like lack of public awareness, unequal distribution of services, unrealistic expectations, lack of skilled staff, extended working hours, etc. is no easy task. These and other constraints can be considered complex cross-cutting problems. This implies that governments and healthcare leaders are required to watch out for the constantly changing external environment, interpreting them to give a sense of direction with a holistic approach.

When new changes are introduced, it is important to work on it as a whole, finding strategies so the ones delivering services (front-line staff, be it doctors, nurses or varied healthcare professionals) and the ones receiving it are both catered to.

It is important to cushion front-line staff who work tirelessly by providing them with job security, a safe environment, financial security and fixed working hours as an overworked health force is not good for the ones providing care and those receiving it.

When staff is under pressure from patient attendants, relatives or friends, there is a dire need to address unacceptable, aggressive behaviours and deal with them appropriately, providing a safe environment so that healthcare staff can deliver the best possible care. Any minor or major incidents should be reviewed and addressed.

Given the pressures that healthcare professionals face in the current scenario, it is important to realise that, at the end of the day, healthcare professionals are also humans who need care and support so that they perform well. A demoralised healthcare team is not a good thing for patients.

Leadership at individual levels

There are different levels at which leadership behaviours play an important role. It is not uncommon that people who are in senior manager roles and the ones who make healthcare delivery-related decisions are far removed from direct care of patients and yet they are the ones who strategise significant changes. The time has come when more medical doctors need to involve themselves in those kinds of roles and this calls for leadership (Kane, 2016).

The leaders at higher positions need to pay heed to staff voice and set clear job descriptions and goals. The teams need to be well supported and there needs to be transparency, especially when it concerns major incidents or errors, auditing and taking appropriate measures to bridge gaps becomes essential (West et al., 2015).

Nurse Leaders

As cited by West et al. (2015), most of the research done in Western countries focuses on nurses and nurse managers. They found strong links between nurse staff job satisfaction and managerial style, retention and turnover; Nurses preferred managers who were facilitative, participative and emotionally intelligent; such styles were associated with lower stress, team cohesion, self-efficacy and higher empowerment. They also found that effective nurse leaders were collaborative, power sharing, flexible and use personal values in promoting high-quality performance.

Medical Leaders

Team effectiveness, providing good patient experience, coordinated care, services, co-designing and organisational development are skills and experiences that clinicians need to possess. Doctors need to train as system leaders (Kane 2016). Doctors and managers have different perspectives on healthcare delivery. As discussed earlier, Indian healthcare basks in its complexity. With private sectors trying to gain a competitive advantage over each other, the hierarchical nature within healthcare systems and people having different priorities at different levels, there is resentment and conflict.

Leadership that pertains to medical leadership is as simple as ensuring change that benefits patient care. The best way to do this is to empower people on the shop-floor the talented doctors and the nurses and allied healthcare professionals who are the real heroes of the healthcare delivery, the ones who work tirelessly for the benefit of patients (Kane 2016). Healthcare is about winning minds and hearts.

If one wants to know where the system is going wrong, it's best to ask patients, interns, postgraduate trainees, duty doctors, consultants and nurses and they will surely know the reasons why the system is failing. These are the people who need to be empowered and the senior leaders should facilitate this change (Kane 2016). There is an urgent need for medical leadership roles and it needs to be taken seriously. There is a need for a new breed of medical leaders not to be mistaken for managerial leaders.

Leadership Within Team

Working towards shared visions and objectives that are achievable, commitment towards a goal, transparency and clarity within the team members are all essential parts of team leadership.

Leaders must ensure that there is shared leadership within the team and the members should be involved in decision-making; constructive debating is necessary to meet challenges and growing demands; members need to be willing to work and collaborate with cross teams. the team needs to regularly discuss and review performance and work towards a positive climate and support each other in good humour (West et al., 2015). The interaction between team members is critical. It is vital to take input from mental health counsellors, nutritionists, nurses, and junior doctors to provide holistic care.

Leadership Within the Organisations

Leadership at higher levels is through creating vision and values. Leaders need to monitor, support, educate, empower and take patient feedback as a yardstick to gauge performance. Heads need to empower staff, motivating them to provide high-quality patient care. It is important to work on strategies that provide work conditions that will nurture a positive work culture (West et al., 2015). Leaders should have forethought in anticipating hurdles and be equipped to handle them.

McFadden et al. (2009), as cited by West et al. (2015), found that the patient safety outcome was linked to CEO leadership style. The research conducted by them revealed that the performance of hospitals depended on the team leadership of the top management; the findings also suggest that effective team leadership was associated with strong and positive clinical governance and a significant drop in the number of patients complaints; furthermore, the feedback rating of both top leads and supervisory leads were positively associated with higher job satisfaction of the staff. It would be exceptionally great for the leaders to develop leadership models in healthcare, working towards and enabling healthcare professionals to deliver quality care. It is also imperative to promote positive and good work cultures and atmospheres so that these professionals provide the best possible outcomes for the patients and the organisations they work for.

National Level Leadership in Health Care

National-level Leadership plays an important role in influencing the healthcare system in the country. Various health bodies have processes and legislations in place. They need to create a vision of providing patient-centred quality care and at the same time provide a platform to healthcare professionals to work towards the set goals.

Challenges

The healthcare system is blighted due to lack of access to healthcare facilities, a shortage of skilled staff such as doctors and paramedical staff and the presence of a predominant number of untrained private practitioners (Sharma, 2015).

Prof. Vikram Patel et al. (2015), suggest that Indian healthcare faces seven challenges:

- The first challenge is that India has a weak primary healthcare sector.

- The second challenge is the unequally skilled human resources.

- The third challenge is the largely unregulated private sector.

- The fourth challenge is the low public spending on healthcare.

- The fifth challenge is a fragmented healthcare information system.

- The sixth challenge is the irrational use and high pricing of technology and drugs.

- The seventh challenge as being weak governance and accountability;

Kasthuri (2018) quotes 5 A's:

- Awareness or the lack of it – Lack of public knowledge about important issues regarding health

- Access or the lack of it – Lack of access to healthcare facilities

- Absence or the human power crisis in healthcare

- Affordability or the cost of healthcare

- Accountability or the lack of it

Innovations That Have Been Sustaining Healthcare Delivery

A Harvard review by Vijay Govindarajan and Ravi Ramamurti (2013) very aptly described the Indian healthcare system and its innovation for survival. Ramamurthy and Govindarajan (2013) identified three trends, what they describe as 'the hub and scope design' having smaller clinics and centres in the periphery/ rural areas and having hubs located in cities where expensive equipment is available, rural areas feeding the hub. The second innovation Govindarajan calls is 'task shifting', where specific tasks are handed down to staff with lower skills and doctors have to handle more complicated cases (Govindarajan, 2013). According to their review, India chronically deals with a shortage of highly skilled doctors. Hospitals have had to maximise their duties and the current situation is still the same. The third is frugality, fanatic about shepherding budget and resources, such as sterilising and reusing surgical instruments (Govindarajan, 2013).

Over time many more establishments have come up, mostly in towns and cities and bills have been passed. The government has introduced many schemes that benefit the populace and the teams at grass roots are doing phenomenal work. However, almost the same strategies mentioned above are being used to meet healthcare demands even today.

Healthcare has become more accessible through telemedicine. Telemedicine can help bridge the gap even in remote areas at least for certain chronic and lifestyle related conditions and mental healthcare. A better strategy should be to use a hybrid approach of in-person consultations and telemedicine follow-ups. Though telemedicine has been there for a long time now, it can be utilised more robustly.

Recently, considerable talk has been about AI and its application in healthcare delivery. This ground-breaking innovation has excellent scope and companies are trying to integrate AI into delivering healthcare and well-being.

Healthcare markets are all talking about how AI can facilitate healthcare delivery. It is still at its infantile stages and will take another few decades for it to integrate itself into the system, aiding healthcare delivery. Technologies such as chatbots are cropping up and there are app-based services but an evidence-based approach is necessary as anything man-made including technology has its drawbacks.

It is essential to remember, though, that something as crucial as health for the very existence and survival of the human race and its well-being will always need a humane, holistic approach with the aid of technology.

Work at hand

According to West et al. (2015), allocating tasks, directing and creating visions, setting organisational goals, encouraging commitment within teams and developing strategies to fulfil the vision are incredibly important aspects of leadership. Leadership works at different levels in the healthcare sector. The primary purpose is to create positive cultures, work towards a better quality of care and cope with the ever-growing demands.

It is phenomenal to realise that the role and context have an impact on leadership characteristics (King's Fund, UK, 2011). The characteristics of leadership vary based on the situation. It has become essential to consider leadership being distributed through both formal and informal roles. Spurgeon et al. cited by King's Fund (2011) note that clinical leaders have taken up responsible and top roles occupying the centre stage. The input from the clinical and managerial leaders, each of different expertise can weigh in to see how problems can be dealt with. There is also a need to consider a contingent view of leadership and consider a vast range of leaders with informal roles in finding solutions to problems that healthcare organisations face.

Given the complexity of the Indian health care system, the hierarchy within organisations both in the public and private sectors, each having its own priorities for achieving certain goals, it may be worthy at this point to say, the private sector has become extremely competitive; one wanting to gain a competitive advantage over the others and this calls for innovation and leadership skills amongst all healthcare professionals. The main goal of the public sector would be to reach out to rural areas, though the process of change will take time and tremendous effort.

Different challenges require different types of leadership; the pressures faced by the Indian healthcare system and the healthcare professionals can be considered as both technical as well as adaptive, both of which call for different leadership approaches. There is also a question of constitutive and perceptual approach; it is thereby important to consider and take into account how a given situation needs to be framed. As Moore & Bennington (2011) suggest, to achieve public value outcomes and expectations, there is a need for strategies in place to address them. This calls for commitment from the government, healthcare governing bodies in the public sector, stakeholders of private healthcare organisations; and addressing resource needs like budget, skilled staff, minimising errors, addressing areas of deficiencies, etc.

In recent times it has become imperative to address the pressures that healthcare professionals face, regarding unrealistic expectations from the public by creating awareness and educating them about the services available to them and regarding health and lifestyle-related issues and their outcomes; preventive and promotive is the way forward. Efforts should be made to address the structural deficiencies in the system and there is a need to create a defined 'healthcare service structure'. The citizens should be made aware of the health services that are available in our country, be it in urban or rural areas, public, private or supported by foundations, NGOs or charities. Efforts should be made to specify the services and their limitations so that people can make informed decisions about the choices that are available to them.

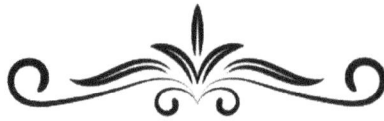

CHAPTER 10

THE PRESENT AND FUTURE OF LEADERSHIP IN HEALTHCARE

*T*here have been many studies conducted internationally regarding the types of effective leadership in healthcare, and they found that transformational leadership theory was the most influential theory guiding healthcare leadership (West et al., 2015). As cited by West et al. (2015), a systematic review conducted by Gilmartin and D'Aunno (2007) examining healthcare leadership found that studies in healthcare provided strong support for transformational leadership theory and identified links with team performance, staff satisfaction, turnover intention and organisational climate. They were of the opinion that effects are stronger when assessed among more junior than senior staff; the positive impact of transformational leadership has also been demonstrated with regards to staff well-being, work-life balance, patient safety, positive nursing outcomes, transparency about errors and staff and patient satisfaction.

The most suitable style for addressing modern complexities and challenges is through transformational leadership (Kouzes & Posner 2007) which involves leading and managing people, working with finite resources, and supporting the physical, emotional and psychological well-being of staff; The 'full leadership range' concept proposed by Bass and Avolio (2011) indicates that transactional and transformational styles may exist within the same individual and their leadership role; this suggests that, to be effective transformational leaders in healthcare, competency development should not just be limited to transformational behaviours but there is also a need to consider transitionally oriented competencies (West et al., 2015). Within healthcare organisations, the role of leaders is quite complex. There is an amalgamation of responsibilities that pertain to both clinical and managerial aspects.

As cited by West et al., (2015), research has reinforced trans-formational leadership at all levels of the organisation because it acknowledges the fact that hospitals and other healthcare organisations have an inverted power structure in which people at the bottom generally have greater influence over decision making on a day-to-day basis than those who are nominally in control at the top (Ham, 2003). Yet, improving transformational leadership will have a positive impact on the performance and satisfaction of the workforce; the positive relationship with this leadership approach has been found to work well for the community, public and private healthcare organisations across the globe and for leaders from all major occupations.

Authentic leadership was also the focus of a small number of studies in health care; this leadership approach emphasises the need to build leader legitimacy through honest relationships with employees by showing value to their contributions and being transparent and ethical; this kind of trust then leads to improvement in performance (West et al., 2015); the nurses who showed authentic leadership towards their managers also showed a greater level of trust, perceptions of quality of care and work engagement (Wong, Laschinger, and Cummings, 2010). Wong and Giallonardo (2013) also found a good relationship between authentic leadership and work-life balance, patient outcomes and managerial trust; moreover, leaders who practice authentic leadership support and encourage nurse empowerment within their roles, this empowerment leads to improved job performance (West et al., 2015).

Gilmartin and D'Aunno (2007), as cited by West at al. (2015), noted at the point they conducted their review that emotional intelligence leadership theory (Goleman, 1995) is relatively neglected in the healthcare literature. There are totally five components to emotional intelligence which are self-awareness, self-regulation, motivation, empathy and social skills (Goldman 2004). According to Keckley (2016), a healthcare policy expert, an organisation that does not take EQ in patient care seriously is prone to low financial and clinical outcomes.

Healthcare is lagging in applying EQ in organisational and patient activities. Research based on patient-physician interactions showed a direct correlation between physicians with low EQ and higher rates of lawsuits, low patient satisfaction and poor outcomes compared to physicians with high EQ (Keckley and Karp, 2016); the research also shows better job satisfaction amongst physicians with higher EQ and improved professional fatigue; emotional intelligence may be highly effective in coping with stress. Healthcare has different dimensions to it, always evolving and faced with pressures and challenges. Managing the stress of 'change management' in healthcare is something that health caregivers must work towards.

Therefore, in conclusion, the evidence through research conducted internationally clearly suggests that transformational leadership and authentic leadership are predictors of quality and performance outcomes within the healthcare system. Though hierarchy, transactional, task-oriented, and aristocratic leadership roles have predominated in the Indian healthcare system, there is a dire need for transformational leaders to bring about innovation and good organisational cultures within the Indian healthcare system.

The system theory, complexity theory and quantum theory have changed the nature and role of leadership (Porter O'Grady & Malloch 2011). There has been a major leap in how leaders are perceived, by shifting from the concept of traits, personality, characteristics or position to a 'set of processes' concerned with deriving action by the staff, towards common goals (Hartley & Benington 2010).

The Newtonian framework which inspired traditional hierarchical control and compartmentalization to manage productivity and people has been replaced by sciences like quantum theory which basks in chaos and complexity and leaders need to have a panoramic view and acknowledge the intersections, relationships and themes to ensure that the organisation runs smoothly (Porter O'Grady & Malloch 2011).

The future will see major transformations in health services and interventions as they become more mobile; and for the deconstruction to be effective, the leaders must equip themselves to lead the change and innovation and to cope with the challenges faced by the organisations (Porter O'Grady & Malloch 2011).

A considerable effort needs to be made to identify the skills, mindsets and behaviour that make a difference between effective and less effective leadership in the healthcare system. Internationally, there have been innumerable number of frameworks to promote managers and leaders in the healthcare sector. Kerr et al. (2006) cited in the King's Fund report (2011) suggest emotional intelligence is a predictor of both leadership and its potential. Hartley and Fletcher (2008) suggest that political awareness of leaders and managers is necessary to be able to deal with the diverse interests of various stakeholders (King's Fund 2011). Both transactional and transformational leadership approaches are necessary to bring about changes in healthcare to achieve desired goals.

Leadership is a dynamic process. Using simple linear models becomes difficult, yet, is important. Hartley & Bennington (2010) suggest public value stream analysis to identify processes by which the system would provide what is valued by the public, which is likely to be quality of care, easy accessibility to health services and affordability. It has become imperative to educate the public about healthcare delivery.

Indian healthcare has many facets to it, scaling from public and private services to everything in between. Digitalisation is gaining popularity and may help in reaching out to remote areas. Research suggests that though telemedicine gained popularity during COVID times, there are pros and cons to it. It is vital to educate the public about the range of services availabe and their limitations so that they make their choices wisely.

It is equally important to empower healthcare organisations, either public or private, to pay heed to the quality of healthcare delivery, which happens by keeping up-to-date through teaching programmes and regular evaluation of service delivery through audits and patient feedback, which are conducted quite regularly to meet accreditations and standards of care.

There is a dire need to hold leadership programs for healthcare professionals to equip them with the skills to deal with today's challenges. Evaluation of these leadership programmes is necessary to know whether these development programmes positively impact the caregivers, organisation and customers. Realistic evaluation by Pawson and Tilley (1997) is one such that addresses the fundamental questions of what works for whom in which circumstances and why that needs to be looked at in depth.

Conclusion

*A*s discussed previously, many things determine healthcare delivery, such as demography, politics, economic constraints, skill sets available, technological advancements, cost of living and governance. Healthcare affordability is an issue for many. There is much scope to provide better primary, secondary and tertiary care where the provision is limited. We must invest in systems and measures that help build the consumers' confidence by providing them with the quality healthcare that they deserve. This calls for formal and informal leadership roles along the echelon of healthcare delivery.

Too often, healthcare organisations are under pressure due to areas concerning resource generation, budget allocation, lack of skilled staff, lack of shared purpose and goals and different priorities at different levels, which are all part and parcel of the private and corporate healthcare sector. It will suffice to say healthcare service has transformed into a healthcare industry. The private sectors work towards gaining a competitive advantage over each other at all times. It is imperative for the corporate stakeholders to breed good work cultures and provide doctors and healthcare professionals with a platform and a safe space to do the best they can. The hope is that many clinical leaders evolve in transforming healthcare delivery.

Studies conducted in the past about leadership and management suggest that leaders and managers face challenges in achieving certain set goals, and financial pressures encourage short-term thinking. It is imperative to develop strategies that will work well with both short-term and long-term goals to provide the best healthcare services.

In the cultures within organisations where there is bullying that stifles leadership potential, there is a lack of senior leaders supporting the leaders below, where healthcare professionals are not given the right platform and a healthy environment to practice, where blame culture is rampant, there is dissatisfaction amongst professionals and this results in poor service delivery. Addressing the above will motivate the staff and healthcare professionals, boost their morale and enhance their performance in providing better services resulting in excellent patient satisfaction and will gain the organisation advantages in all prospects.

Though a well-placed hierarchy and a controlled structure with positive bureaucracy are required for high governance and leadership, there is also a need for some innovation and flexibility to tackle issues at the local level and to solve pressures the healthcare systems face. The input of professionals at the frontline of healthcare delivery and those holding the fort needs to be acknowledged to create a sound healthcare system.

The scope of co-creation approaches with different stakeholders can be widened when it comes to private establishments. It becomes essential for policymakers and managers to lead the change process beyond traditional barriers. However, one should realise that patient-centred quality care should be the ultimate shared vision and the rest, be it profitability, productivity or competitive advantage will naturally follow.

There is a need for long-term strategies while paying attention to patients' and employees' everyday experiences. There is an urgency and measures must be taken in the private and public healthcare sectors. Clear goals and formal and informal leadership roles must be defined. It is essential to ensure that these leaders don't become another part of the existing complexity within an organisation or the system but bring about the required transformational change. The 'change' process will have to overcome obstacles such as a lack of strategic responsibility for their implementation which makes it a challenging task.

References

Ackerman, L. (1997). *Development, transition or transformation: the question of change in organizations.* London: Oxford Publishers.

Ad Hoc Advisory group., (2006). Differentiating Audit, Service Evaluation and Research Available at: http://www.shef.ac.uk/polopoly_fs/1.158539!/file/AuditorResearch.pdf

Adair, J.E. (1973). "Action-Centered Leadership". McGraw-Hill, London.

Al- Sawai, A. (2013). Leadership of Healthcare Professionals, Where do we stand? Oman Medical Journal, Available at https://www.ncbi.nlm.nih.gov/pmc/articles/PMC3725246/

American Psychiatric Association. (2022). *Diagnostic and statistical manual of mental disorders* (5th ed., text rev.). https://doi.org/10.1176/appi.books.9780890425787

Armstrong, M. (2009). Armstrong's Handbook of Human Resource Management Practice#

Bass, B. M., & Avolio, B. J. (1993). Transformational leadership: A response to critiques. M. M. Chemers & R. Ayman (Eds.), Leadership theory and research: Perspectives and directions San Diego, CA: Academic Press

Barr, J., (2011). Leadership in Health Care, SAGE.

Bellot, J. (2011). Defining and assessing organisational culture *Nursing Forum* Available at: http://onlinelibrary.wiley.com/doi/10. 1111/j.1744-6198.2010.00207.x/abstract?userIsAuthenticated= false&deniedAccessCustomisedMessage=

Benington J., Moore M. H. (2011). *Public value : theory and practice.* Palgrave Macmillan.

Burns, J. M. (1978). Leadership, Harper and Row, New York.

Buchbinder, B. S., Shanks, H. N. (2009). Introduction to healthcare management, Jones and Bartlett Publishing

Bryman, A., Collinson, D., Grint, K., Jackson, B., Uhl-Bien, M. (2011). The Sage Handbook of Leadership, SAGE

Cattell, R. B. (1965). The Scientific Analysis of Personality Emotional Intelligence depends on more than physician behavior, Available at: http://www.hhnmag.com/articles/7261-emotional-intelligence-depends-on-more-than-physicianbehavior?utm_campaign=051716& utm_medium=email&utm_source=hhndaily&utm_source= hhndaily&utm_medium=email&utm_campaign=051716&eid= 333956129&bid=1406734

Chaidi, I., & Drigas, A. (2022). "Theories - models of emotional intelligence". Scientific Electronic Archives. Researchgate

Available at: https://www.researchgate.net/publication/365886008_ Theories_-_models_of_emotional_intelligence

Commission Resources (1999). Florence nightingale: Measuring hospital care outcomes, Joint Commission Resources, Oak Brook, Illinois

Degeling, P., Kennedy, J., & Hill, M. (2001). Mediating the cultural boundaries between medicine, nursing and management-the central challenge in hospital reform. *Health Services Management Research*, 14(1), 36-48. Available at: http://hsm.sagepub.com/content/14/1/36.short

Dossey, B. M., Beck, D. M., Selanders L., Attewell A. (2004). Florence Nightingale today: Healing, leadership, global action, American Nurses Association, Silver Spring, Maryland.

Drucker, F. P., (1954). The practice of Management, The Wall Street Journal.

Ferlie, E., & Pettigrew, A. (2005). Managing Through Networks: Some Issues and Implications for the NHS. British Journal of Management. Available at: https://www.researchgate.net/publication/229596361_Managing_Through_Networks_Some_Issues_and_Implications_for_the_NHS/citation/download

Fiedler, F. E. (1958). Leader attitudes and group effectiveness. University Illinois Press.

Fleishman, E. A. (1953). The description of supervisory behavior. Journal of Applied Psychology, 37(1), 1–6. https://doi.org/10.1037/h0056314.

Freud, S. (1912). The dynamics of transference, Word press. Available @ https://readingsinpsych.files.wordpress.com/2009/08/freud-dynamics-of-transference.pdf

Freud. (1931). "Libidinal Types", The Standard Edition of the Complete Psychological Works of Sigmund Freud, vol. XXI, London: The Hogarth Press and the Institute of Psychoanalysis.

Ginter, M. P., Duncan J. W., Swayne E. L. (2013). The Strategic Management of Health Care Organization. Jossey-Bass.

Gilmartin, M.J., and D'Aunno, T. A. (2007). Leadership Research in Healthcare: A Review and Roadmap. The Academy of Management Annals. Available at: https://doi.org/10.1080/078559813

Greenleaf, R. (2008). The Servant as Leader. Westfield, IN: The Greenleaf Centre for Servant Leadership.

Greenleaf, R. (1972). *The Institution as a Servant* . Westfield, IN: The Greenleaf Centre for Servant Leadership.

Govindarajan, V., Ramamurthi, R. (2013). India's Secret to Low-Cost Health Care, Harvard Business Review. Available at: https://hbr.org/2013/10/indias-secret-to-low-cost-health-care

Greig, G., Entwistle, V. A., Beech, N. (2012), Addressing complex healthcare problems in diverse settings: insights from activity theory. Pub Med. Available at https://pubmed.ncbi.nlm.nih.gov/21420212/

Gupta, I., and Chowdhury, S., (2016). "Urban Concerns and Their Impact on Health in India," in K. Eggleston (ed.), Policy Challenges from Demographic Change in China and India. Available at: at https://www.worldwidejournals.com/international-journal-of-scientific-research-(IJSR)/recent_issues_pdf/2018/October/October_2018_1538384468__08.pdf

Gupta, I., Bhatia, M. (2016).The Indian Healthcare system, International Healthcare system Profiles, The Common Wealth Fund. Available at: http://international.commonwealthfund.org/countries/india/

Hart, E., & Hazelgrove, J. (2001). Understanding the organisational context for adverse events in the health services: the role of cultural censorship. *Quality in Health Care*, *10*(4), 257-262. Available at: http://qualitysafety.bmj.com/content/10/4/257.short

Hartley, J., Benington, J. (2010). Leadership for Healthcare, Bristol Policy Press.

Hartley, J., Benington, J. (2011), Recent trends in Leadership, Thinking and Action in the public and voluntary services sector. King's Fund Available at https://www.kingsfund.org.uk/sites/default/files/recent-trends-in-leadership-thinking-action-in-public-voluntary-service-sectors-jean-hartley-john-benington-kings-fund-may-2011.pdf

Iles, V., Sutherland, K. (2001). Organisational change: A review for health care managers, professionals and researches, National institute of health research (NIHR) Available at: http://www.netscc.ac.uk/hsdr/files/project/SDO_FR_08-1001-001_V01.pdf

Indian Healthcare Industry Analysis, (2017)., IBEF Available at: https://www.ibef.org/industry/healthcare-presentation

Jasper, M., Jumma M. (2005). Effective healthcare Leadership, Blackwell publishing limited.

Johnson, G., Scholes, K., Whittington, R. (2008). Exploring Corporate Strategy, 8 th Edition, Prentice Hall.

Kane, B. (2016). Why is Medical Leadership important in Healthcare, King's Fund Available at: https://www.kingsfund.org.uk/blog/2016/01/why-medical-leadership-important-health-service

Kasthuri A. (2018). Challenges to Healthcare in India - The Five A's. Indian J Community Med. Pubmed Central. Available at: https://www.ncbi.nlm.nih.gov/pmc/articles/PMC6166510/

Karla, N. R. (2011). A Doctor par Excellence, The Hindu. Available at: http://www.thehindu.com/opinion/open-page/a-doctor-par-excellence/article2153732.ece

Keckley, P., and Karp, M. (2016). Emotional Intelligence depends on more than Physical Behavior, H&HN, AHA Publication. Available at: http://www.hhnmag.com/articles/7261-emotional-intelligence-depends-on-more-than-physician-behavior

Kennett, M.,= (2002). Management Today, Haymarket Business publications.

Kellerman, B. (1986). Political Leadership: A source book, University of Pittsburgh Press.

Kets de Vries M.,& Miller, D. (1984), Narcissism and Leadership: An object relations perspective, INSEAD, Fontainebleau, France. Available at: https://flora.insead.edu/fichiersti_wp/Inseadwp1985/85-19.pdf

Kets de Vries, M., Cheak, A. (2014). Psychodynamic Approach. SSRN Electronic Journal. 10.2139/ssrn.2456594. Available at: https://sites.insead.edu/facultyresearch/research/doc.cfm?did=54942

King's Fund (2011), The Future of Leadership and Management report Available at: https://www.kingsfund.org.uk/sites/files/kf/Future-of-leadership-and-management-NHS-May-2011-The-Kings-Fund.pdf

Kirkpatick, S. A., and E. A. Locke. (1991). "Leadership: do traits matter?" The executive. ResearchGate. Available at: https://www.researchgate.net/publication/262082812_Leadership_Do_Traits_Matter

Kotter, J. (1996). Leading Change, Boston: Harvard Business School Press

Kotter, J. & Cohen, D., (2002), The Heart Of Change, Boston: Harvard Business School Press.

Kouzes, J. M., & Posner, B. Z. (1987). The leadership challenge: How to get extraordinary things done in organizations.Jossey-Bass.

Lewin, K. (1952). Field theory in social science. 1st ed. London: Tavistock Publications.

Madanchian, M.,Hussein, N., & Noordin, F., Taherdoost, H., (2016). Leadership Theories; an Overview of Early Stages. Available at: https://www.researchgate.net/publication/305323677_Leadership_Theories_an_Overview_of_Early_Stages/citation/download

Malloch, K., Porter O' Grady T. (2009). Innovation Leadership, Creating the Landscape for Healthcare, Jones and Bartlett Publishers.

Martin, V., Charlesworth, H. E. (2010). Managing in Health and Social Care

Mcgregor, D., Douglas mcgregor's XY theory, managing an X theory boss, and William Ouchi's theory Z. Available at http://www.businessballs.com/mcgregor.htm

Ministry of Health and Family welfare (2015). Department of Health and family welfare Available at: https://main.mohfw.gov.in/documents/publications/annual-report-department-health-family-welfare-year-2015-16/annual-report-department-health-family-welfare-year-2015-16

Ministry of Health and Family welfare (2016). Department of Health and family welfare Available at: https://main.mohfw.gov.in/ annual-report-department-health-and-family-welfare--2016-17

Mintzberg, H., Ahlstrand, B., Lampel, J. (2009). Strategic Safari, The Free Press, New York.

Mintzberg H. (1989). Meintzberg on Management, The Free Press

Mitra. P., Fluyau, D.,(2023). Narcissistic Personality Disorder. StatPearls [Internet]. Treasure Island Available at: https://www.ncbi.nlm.nih.gov/ books/NBK556001/

Mullins L J. (2005). Management and Organisational Behaviour.

National Health Policy. (2017) available at https://www.nhp.gov.in// NHPfiles/national_health_policy_2017.pdf

National Health Policy Draft, 2015, (2014) available at https://www. mygov.in/frontendgeneral/pdf/draft-national-health-policy.pdf

Northouse, P, G. (2011). Introduction to Leadership concepts and Practices, Sage publication

NHS England, Discomfort Zone, Online Library of quality, service improvement and redesign tools. Available at: https://www.england. nhs.uk/wp-content/uploads/2022/01/qsir-discomfort-zone.pdf

Ozcan, A. Y. (2009). Quantitative Methods in Healthcare Management, techniques and applications, second edition, Jossey-Bass.

Patel, V., Parikh R., Nandraj S., Balasubramaniam P., Narayan, K, Paul K. V., S. K. A Kumar., Chatterjee, M., Reddy K. S.(2015). Assuring health coverage for all in India. Lancet, Available at: http://www.thelancet. com/journals/lancet/article/PIIS0140-6736(15)00955-1/fulltext

Pawson, R., Tilley, N. (1997). Realistic Evaluation, SAGE Publication Ltd.

Peters TJ., Waterman RH. (1982). In *Search of Excellence: Lessons from America's Best - Run Companies*. New York: Harper and Row, Available at: http://www.jstor.org/stable/2393015

Plesk, E, P., Wilson T. (2001). Complexity, leadership and management in healthcare organisations BMJ group Available at: http://www.bmj.com/content/323/7315/746.1?tab=responses

Porter, O'-Grady, T., Malloch, K. (2011). Quantum Leadership Advancing Innovation, Transforming healthcare, third edition, Jones & Bartlett publishing.

Porter, L. W., & McLaughlin, G. B. (2006). Leadership and the Organizational Context: Like the Weather? The Leadership Quarterly, 17, 559-576.

Rollinson, D. (2008). Organisational Behavior and Analysis. An Integrated approach, 4th Edn. Pearson Education Limited.

Schien, E. H. (2004). Organisational Culture and Leadership, 3rd edition, Jossey Bass

Reynolds, M. (2014). The Discomfort Zone: How Leaders Turn Difficult Conversations into Breakthroughs, San Francisco: Berrett-Koehler

Schein, E. H. (2010). *Organisational culture and leadership* (Vol. 2). John Wiley & Sons. Available at: https://books.google.com.pk/books?hl=en&lr=&id=kZH6AwTwZV8C&oi=fnd&pg=PR9&dq=organisational+culture&ots=9nd6nGtzRd&sig=rA8tmzEOOglLd6Km5pB19rNJOlA

Schein, E. H. (1995). The Role of the Founder in Creating Organizational Culture. Family Business Review, 8(3), 221–238. https://doi.org/10.1111/j.1741-6248.1995.00221.x

Schien, E. H. (2009). The Corporate Culture Survival Guide, Jossey Bass, Hoboken.

Sheingold, H. B., Hahn, J. (2014). The History of Healthcare quality, the first 100 years, 1860-1960, The Gorge Washington University Health Sciences Research Commons, Nursing Faculty Publications, Available at http://hsrc.himmelfarb.gwu.edu/cgi/viewcontent.cgi?article=1111&context=son_nurs_facpubs

Sharma C. (2015). India still struggles with rural doctor shortage, Lancet, available at: http://www.thelancet.com/journals/lancet/article/PIIS0140-6736(15)01231-3/fulltext

Stogdill, M. R. (1948). Personal Factors Associated with Leadership: A Survey of the Literature. Journal of Psychology. Available at: https://doi.org/10.1080/00223980.1948.9917362

Stogdill, M. R. (1963). *Manual for the Leader Behavior Description Questionnaire – Form XII: An Experimental Revision* (PDF). Fisher College of Business, Ohio State University.

Strock, M. J. (2016). Serve to Lead, your 21st century Leadership System. Available at: http://servetolead.org/21st-century-leadership-vs-20th-century-leadership/

Stoller, K. J., Goodall A., Baker A., (2016), Why the best Hospitals are managed by doctors, Harvard review, Available at: https://hbr.org/2016/12/why-the-best-hospitals-are-managed-by-doctors

The NHS Confederation (2007). The Challenges of leadership in the NHS Available at: http://www.nhsconfed.org/Publications/Documents/The%20challenges%20of%20leadership%20in%20the%20NHS.pdf

The NHS Confederation (2007), Priority Setting: An Overview, Available at: http://www.nhsconfed.org/~/media/Confederation/Files/Publications/Documents/Priority%20setting%20an%20overview.pdf

Sawicki, P., Bastian, H. (2008). German health care: A bit of Bismarck plus more science. BMJ. Available at: https://www.bmj.com/content/337/bmj.a1997.full

Tabish, S. A. (2000). Hospital & Health Services Administration: Principles & Practice, First Edition, Publisher: Oxford University Press.

Turnbull, J. (2011). Leadership in Context, Lessons from New Leadership theory and current leadership development practice (online) Available at: www.Kingsfund.org.uk\leadershipcommission

Weick, K. E., & Quinn, R. E. (1999). Organizational change and development. *Annual Review of Psychology, 50,* 361–386. https://doi.org/10.1146/annurev.psych.50.1.361

West, M., Armit, K., Loewenthal, L., Eckert, R., West, T., Lee, A. (2015), Leadership and Leadership Development in Healthcare: The Evidence base, King's Fund Available at: https://www.kingsfund.org.uk/sites/files/kf/field/field_publication_file/leadership-leadership-development-health-care-feb-2015